FUNDAMENTALS OF NURSING - NCLEX-RN EXAM REVIEW:

349 Practice Questions with Detailed Rationales
Explaining Correct & Incorrect Answer Choices

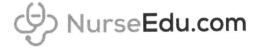

Disclaimer:

Although the author and publisher have made every effort to ensure that the information in this book was correct at press time, the author and publisher do not assume and hereby disclaim any liability to any party for any loss, damage, or disruption caused by errors or omissions, whether such errors or omissions result from negligence, accident, or any other cause.

This book is not intended as a substitute for the medical advice of physicians. The reader should regularly consult a physician in matters relating to their health and particularly with respect to any symptoms that may require diagnosis or medical attention.

NCLEX®, NCLEX®-RN, and NCLEX®-PN are registered trademarks of the National Council of State Boards of Nursing, Inc. They hold no affiliation with this product.

Some images within this book are either royalty-free images, used under license from their respective copyright holders, or images that are in the public domain.

ISBN: 978-1-952914-10-2

FREE BONUS

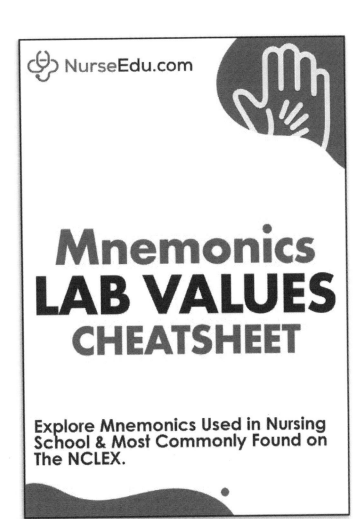

FREE Download – Just Visit:

NurseEdu.com/bonus

TABLE OF CONTENTS

CHAPTER 1:

NCLEX-RN – FUNDAMENTALS: BASIC CARE AND COMFORT/PAIN MANAGEMENT

Multiple Choice

1. The nurse encourages a patient with a history of heart failure to reduce energy expenditure by alternating activity and rest. Which nursing process phase is this?

    A. Diagnosis
    B. Planning
    C. Implementation
    D. Evaluation

Rationale:

Correct answer: C

Teaching a patient about alternating activity and rest is a component of patient education, which falls into the implementation phase. This is an example of putting an individualized plan into action. Other components of implementation include assisting with hygienic care, promoting physical comfort, supporting respiratory and elimination functions, facilitating ingestion of food/fluids, managing the patient's surroundings, promoting a therapeutic relationship, and carrying out other therapeutic nursing activities.

A is incorrect because diagnosis is identifying the problem. When choosing the diagnoses for a particular client, the nurse must first identify commonalities among the assessment data collected. Categorization of related data reveals the existence of a problem and the need for nursing intervention. The patient's identified problems are then defined in the nursing diagnoses.

B is incorrect because planning is creating an individualized plan. The planning phase includes assigning priorities to the diagnoses, specifying the goals, identifying the interventions/outcomes, documenting the plan, and communicating the plan to nursing staff.

D is incorrect because evaluation is assessing patient response to an individualized plan.

*Remember that dividing the nursing process into separate steps is actually artificial. The process functions as an integrated whole, with the steps being interrelated, interdependent, and recurrent.

2. The nurse on the medical-surgical unit is interested in implementing evidence-based practice. The nurse knows when evidence-based practice is utilized:

    A. National health agencies create clinical practice guidelines that must be used.
    B. Findings from randomized trials are used to plan care.
    C. Clinical decision-making and nursing judgment are used to find which evidence works for each specific situation in clinical practice.
    D. Nursing interventions are statistically analyzed by a nurse in relation to patient outcomes to discover evidence for appropriate patient interventions.

Rationale:

Correct answer: C

Evidence-based practice is based on evidence from nurses working with actual patients to find the best interventions for the best outcomes. It is through this evidence that nurses develop and improve their practice to achieve even greater patient outcomes. It is imperative that nurses continue to learn and improve their skills and use updated techniques as technology changes and patients have increasing acuity.

A is incorrect because clinical practice guidelines are not consistently updated or based on current evidence. National health agencies such as the Department of Health & Human Services, Department of Labor (which includes OSHA), and non-governmental agencies (such as JCAHO) do influence nursing practice but are not essential to evidence-based practice.

B is incorrect because randomized trials are not consistently pertinent to each patient's illness, and findings from trials cannot be utilized to shape care for all patient problems. Randomized trials are carefully planned experiments that introduce treatment or exposure to study the effect on actual patients. They may be used to shape evidence-based practice, but not necessarily.

D is incorrect because evidence is based on nursing practice globally, not on one nurse's practice.

3. New nurses in orientation are learning about completion of incident reports. Which of the following incidents would require an incident report be filed?

    A. Medication given 30 minutes before scheduled time

    B. Patient belongings lost when transferred to their hospital room

    C. Frayed electrical cord on an IV pump

    D. Medication order missing route of administration

Rationale:

Correct answer: B.

Any time a patient's belongings are lost an incident report must be filed. This can help identify people and departments involved, ways to prevent the occurrence in the future, and even help in locating belongings.

A is incorrect because administering a medication 30 minutes before scheduled time is not an error. Nurses are generally required to administer *scheduled* meds within 30 minutes before or after they are scheduled.

C is incorrect because this equipment should be taken out of service and the biomedical department notified, but this situation does not require an incident report to be completed.

D is incorrect because the healthcare provider can be notified and the order clarified. An incident report is not needed.

*Remember: The client's chart is client-focused. The incident report is incident-focused. In the incident report, the nurse must include the time and place of the incident and must objectively describe what happened, who was involved, how the client responded, actions that were performed at the time of the event, and the name of the physician who was notified.

4. A nurse enters a patient's room to deliver medications that are due and discovers the patient is in the bathroom. Which of the following actions by the nurse is appropriate?

    A. Place the medication on the bedside table

    B. Place the medication on the bedside table and tell the patient not to forget to take them

    C. Ask the patient to call when out of the bathroom and give the medications at that time

    D. Ask the patient to call when out of the bathroom and leave the medications on the bedside table

Rationale:

Correct answer: C

The nurse should return when the patient is available to take the medications so the nurse can verify the medications have been taken. The nurse should never leave medications on the bedside table.

Remember, the rights of medication administration:

1. Right patient: use two identifiers
2. Right medication: check the med label AND the order
3. Right dose: check the order, perform calculation if necessary, and refer to the drug book if needed to confirm safe dose.
4. Right route: is the route appropriate? Can the patient safely take the med by this route?
5. Right time: check the frequency, confirm that the right dose was given at the right time, and check when the last dose was given.
6. Right documentation: document AFTER giving the meds. Include any pertinent details, such as the injection site.
7. Right reason: confirm the rationale for the ordered medication. Why is the patient getting it?
8. Right response: be sure that the drug led to the desired effect. Monitor for side effects or adverse reactions after giving it.

A, B, C are incorrect because medications should never be left in the patient room.

5. The nurse is preparing to perform a focused assessment of the patient's abdomen. Which of the following choices is the correct order in which the focused assessment is performed?

   A. Palpation, Auscultation, Inspection, Percussion
   B. Inspection, Palpation, Percussion, Auscultation
   C. Percussion, Palpation, Inspection, Auscultation
   D. Inspection, Auscultation, Percussion, Palpation

Rationale:

Correct answer: D

When performing an abdominal assessment, inspection and auscultation should be performed prior to percussion and palpation because the last two techniques will alter bowel sounds. Inspection is looking at the appearance of the abdomen while the patient is lying supine, with their arms by their side, and head resting on a pillow. (If the neck is flexed, abdominal muscles may become flexed, and this can alter the appearance during assessment.).

Auscultation is performed over all four quadrants. Consider, are bowel sounds present? What are the quality and quantity of the bowel sounds? Note any regional differences among the four quadrants. Percussion is performed by the fingers to test for dullness (solid mass) and tympany (air or gas).

Palpation is performed to discover any pain or tenderness. When palpating, apply slow, steady pressure and avoid sharp movements that may cause discomfort.

A is incorrect because bowel sounds will be altered by palpating before auscultating.

B is incorrect because bowel sounds will be altered by palpating and percussing before auscultating. Note: This IPPA sequence is the correct sequence for assessing other body systems, but not correct in the abdominal assessment.

C is incorrect because bowel sounds will be altered by performing the auscultation last.

6. A patient is in the clinic with complaints of "not feeling well." The nurse knows the patient's primary defense against infection is:

   A. Fever
   B. Intact skin
   C. Inflammation
   D. Lethargy

Rationale:

Correct answer: B.

The primary defense from infection is intact skin. Breaks in the skin allow a route for infection to invade.

A is incorrect because fever is a secondary defense against infection. Fever is significant when above 100.4°F or 38°C.

C is incorrect because inflammation is a secondary defense against infection. Inflammation produces redness, pain, swelling, and warmth as a result of infection, irritation, or injury. The body heals during the inflammatory process as leukocytes and proteins migrate to the area in order to fight infection and repair damage.

D is incorrect because lethargy is not a defense against infection. Lethargy can be a symptom of infection.

7. The nurse on the medical unit is caring for a patient who does not speak English, and the nurse does not understand the patient's language. Which of the following is most appropriate for the nurse to do when speaking with the patient?

   A. Have the patient's wife translate
   B. Speak using medical terminology to avoid misunderstanding

C. Keep in mind translation is more important than nonverbal communication

D. Have a certified medical interpreter translate

Rationale:

Correct answer: D

Medical interpreters are certified in translation for scenarios like this. Rigorous training and testing is performed before becoming a medical interpreter, so this is the best way to interpret for a patient and prevent mistakes and misunderstandings.

A is incorrect because family members are emotionally involved in a situation and cannot necessarily remain neutral. A family member may try to interpret in a way to persuade the patient. The family member is not a professionally trained interpreter and we cannot assume they have a knowledge and understanding of medical terminology.

B is incorrect because medical terminology will not prevent misunderstandings as these words are not well understood.

C is incorrect because nonverbal communication is almost as important as the words and translations themselves.

8. The nurse is completing the preoperative checklist for a patient scheduled for surgery. In reviewing the chart, the nurse finds the consent has not been signed by the patient. When the patient starts asking questions regarding the surgery, what is the next action the nurse should take?

    A. Have the patient sign the consent
    B. Tell the patient all questions will be answered by the surgeon before the anesthesiologist administers anesthetic
    C. Contact the surgeon to inform them the patient has questions regarding the procedure
    D. Answer all the patient's questions

Rationale:

Correct answer: C

Before any invasive procedure, the surgeon must inform the patient of what the procedure entails, the purpose for the procedure, and the potential risks associated with that procedure before the consent is signed by the patient. (Hence the term "informed consent.") If the consent has not been signed and the patient has questions, the healthcare provider has not reviewed the procedure and risks involved and needs to do so before the procedure.

A is incorrect because the patient has questions and has not been informed by the surgeon. The nurse does not obtain the signed consent. The nurse's duty is to witness the explanation and sign as a witness that the client understands the procedure.

B is incorrect because this patient has not been informed about the procedure at all and passing it off to the surgeon does not promote patient-centered care. The nurse should not wait until the patient is in the OR (or procedure room) to get consent. Consent should be obtained before the client is transferred within the facility. This answer choice is also non-therapeutic as it dismisses the client's concerns.

D is incorrect because the nurse's duty is to answer questions (within the nurse's knowledge base) *after* the consent has been signed. It is the health care provider's responsibility to review the consent and risks.

9. The nurse is caring for a patient who had an endoscopic total hysterectomy and is now experiencing urinary retention. The nurse is preparing to contact the healthcare provider using SBAR (situation background assessment recommendation). Which of the following questions is a part of SBAR communication?

    A. "Could you tell me what I need to do?"
    B. "What do you need to know about the patient?"
    C. "I believe the patient needs a urinary catheter."
    D. "Why do you think the patient is unable to urinate?"

Rationale:

Correct answer: C

Making a recommendation to the healthcare provider is part of SBAR.

A is incorrect because asking the healthcare provider what to do is unprofessional, not appropriate, and not part of SBAR.

B is incorrect because the nurse should be prepared to provide the patient's history pertinent to the current situation.

D is incorrect because asking the healthcare provider what the contributing factors are is not appropriate and not part of SBAR.

The SBAR sequence offers hospitals and healthcare facilities a way to standardize communication related to patient hand-off, transfers, and requests for physicians' orders.

The following is an example of how the nurse could effectively use SBAR in this patient situation:

> *Situation*: "Mrs. Jones is experiencing urinary retention."

Background: "She had an endoscopic total hysterectomy.

Assessment: Her vital signs have been stable today. She is taking PO fluids but has had no urine output in the last five hours. Her bladder is distended."

Recommendation: "I recommend that you see her and we insert an indwelling urinary Foley catheter and measure urine output every two hours."

10. A patient is recovering from a total abdominal hysterectomy. When assessed by the nurse eight hours after the procedure, which of the following would the nurse identify as an early sign of shock?

   A. Restlessness
   B. Warm, dry skin that is pale
   C. Heart rate of 115 bpm
   D. Urine output 50 mL/hr

Rationale:

Correct answer: A

Early signs of shock include restlessness, anxiousness, nervousness, and irritability. This is due to the sympathetic nervous system release of epinephrine, which also decreases perfusion to the skin causing pallor, coolness, and clamminess. Other signs of shock include hypotension and confusion.

B is incorrect because in shock the skin is pale, cool, and clammy.

C is incorrect because increased heart rate is a late sign of shock.

D is incorrect because the urine output is within normal limits and is not a significant finding related to shock. In shock, the nurse would expect to observe decreased urine output.

11. A patient is admitted to the emergency room complaining of shortness of breath. The nurse knows the patient will be evaluated for hypoxia and anticipates the healthcare provider ordering which test?

   A. Complete blood cell count (CBC)
   B. Sputum culture
   C. Hemoglobin (Hgb)
   D. Arterial blood gas (ABG)

Rationale:

Correct answer: D

An ABG evaluates gas exchange in the lungs, which will provide the needed information regarding oxygenation status. An arterial blood gas reveals pH, carbon dioxide and oxygen partial pressures, bicarbonate level (HCO_3-), and pH.

- Remember, the normal values reflected in an ABG:

  pH normal = 7.35-7.45

  (Carbon Dioxide) CO_2 normal = 35-45

  (Oxygen) O_2 normal = 80-100

  (Bicarbonate) HCO_3 normal = 22-26

- Low pH (less than 7.35) = acidosis

  High CO_2 (greater than 45) = respiratory acidosis

  Low bicarb (less than 22) = metabolic acidosis

- High pH (greater than 7.45) = basic (alkalosis)

  Low CO_2 (less than 35) = respiratory alkalosis

  High bicarb (greater than 26) = metabolic alkalosis

A is incorrect because a CBC is not a test that specifically evaluates shortness of breath.

- CBC measures total red blood cell count, white blood cell count, differential WBC count, hematocrit, hemoglobin, mean corpuscular volume, mean corpuscular hemoglobin, and mean corpuscular hemoglobin concentration.

B is incorrect because a sputum culture is performed to diagnose infection of the lungs. This question does not give us any information about the pulmonary assessment or accumulation of secretions in the lungs. A sputum culture will confirm which, if any, microorganisms are present in the lungs, but will not help us evaluate hypoxia.

C is incorrect because, although hemoglobin can reflect the ability of the body's erythrocytes to carry oxygen, it will not be as helpful in evaluating shortness of breath and hypoxia as an ABG.

- Normal Hgb = male 13-18, female 12-16, child 11-12.5.

12. Emergency medical services brings an unconscious adult in to the emergency room.

    When the nurse performs a rapid assessment, the location to check the pulse is:

    A. Radial

    B. Brachial

    C. Femoral

D. Carotid

Rationale:

Correct answer: D

Rapid assessment of an unconscious adult patient begins with checking circulation, which is checked at the carotid artery. If a patient is hypotensive (decreased blood pressure), the most likely place to be able to feel a pulse is the carotid artery.

A is incorrect because circulatory compromise and hypotension may make a radial pulse difficult to palpate.

B is incorrect because the brachial pulse is palpated for rapid assessment of an infant.

C is incorrect because the most effective way to check an adult's pulse is the carotid artery which is closer to the heart and more superficial than the femoral artery.

13. A patient is admitted to the medical-surgical unit with methicillin-resistant staphylococcus aureus (MRSA) of a wound. The nurse initiates contact precautions, which includes use of which of the following?

    A. Clean gown and gloves
    B. N-95 respirator
    C. Biohazard bin placed in the room
    D. Negative airflow room

Rationale:

Correct answer: A

Contact isolation requires all people entering the room to follow standard precautions in addition to wearing a clean (not sterile) gown and gloves. Other diseases that require contact precautions include the following: norovirus, rotavirus, and *Clostridium difficile*. Additionally, patients with draining wounds, uncontrolled secretions, pressure ulcers, generalized rash, and ostomy bags/tubes also warrant contact precautions.

B is incorrect because N-95 respirators are for patients on airborne precautions. Diseases that require airborne precautions include the following: measles, chickenpox, shingles, tuberculosis, and smallpox.

C is incorrect because linen and trash for this patient are not considered biohazardous.

D is incorrect because negative airflow rooms are for patients on airborne precautions. The negative pressure allows air to enter into the room, but air is evacuated from the room and expelled outside of the healthcare facility to prevent spread of airborne contaminants within the building's ventilation system.

14. A patient in the medical-surgical unit tells the nurse they haven't had a bowel movement in two days. What is the first intervention the nurse should implement?

    A. Review the patient's medical record to determine normal bowel pattern
    B. Offer prune juice with every meal
    C. Call the healthcare provider to request an order for stool softener
    D. Increase the patient's oral fluid intake

Rationale:

Correct answer: A

Bowel patterns can vary greatly in adults: three BMs weekly up to three BMs daily is considered within normal range. Several factors can influence normal bowel patterns, including surgery, stress, and opioid medications. The nurse should review the medical record to determine the patient's normal bowel patterns prior to hospitalization.

B is incorrect because prune juice at every meal can lead to diarrhea. It is more important to determine the patient's baseline bowel routine.

C is incorrect because a stool softener may not be indicated if this is the patient's normal bowel pattern. It is always best to look for a nursing answer that is non-pharmacologic.

D is incorrect because we do not yet have any information about the amount of fluids the patient is currently taking. Increasing PO fluids could lead to fluid volume overload.

15. A 40-year-old patient in the clinic tells the nurse they have frequent constipation. The patient has taken steps to remedy the constipation but would like to prevent it with a bowel-training program. Which of the following is of greatest concern to the nurse?

    A. The patient does not eat any fruits and vegetables
    B. The patient drinks 2 liters of water daily
    C. The patient exercises 3 to 4 days per week
    D. The patient's home recently tested positive for lead

Rationale:

Correct answer: D

Lead poisoning can cause constipation. This is the greatest concern for the nurse at this time. The patient will need their blood to be tested for lead, and other people living in the home will need to be assessed as well.

A is incorrect because although fruits and vegetables (high in fiber) will help prevent constipation, it is more important to address the pathological cause of the constipation.

B is incorrect because adequate fluids will help with constipation. Drinking 2 liters of water daily provides most average adults with their daily fluid needs.

C is incorrect because exercise will help with constipation. Exercising 3-5 times per week is optimal for average adults.

16. A patient appears anxious about an upcoming procedure. Which of the following responses by the nurse will reduce this patient's anxiety?

    A. "Don't worry. It will be fine."
    B. "Read this pamphlet about the procedure and let me know if you have questions."
    C. "I will turn on some music for you."
    D. "Would you like to talk about what's bothering you?"

Rationale:

Correct answer: D

Anxiety is common before medical procedures. The patient may feel helpless, isolated, or insecure. Encouraging the patient to talk about their feelings can reduce anxiety and helps the nurse be supportive by developing goals with the patient for some sense of control. This is the response that displays therapeutic communication.

A is incorrect because it ignores the patient's feelings and prevents patient-centered care. Saying, "don't worry," is non-therapeutic because it dismisses the patient's anxiety.

B is incorrect because it is *passing the buck* and does not promote the nurse-client relationship.

C is incorrect because it does not address the patient's anxiety. Distraction is not a therapeutic technique for addressing anxiety.

17. A patient is admitted to the cardiac unit after myocardial infarction (MI). The patient tells the nurse they don't want their spouse to know what happened. What is the best response by the nurse?

    A. "I have to tell your spouse what happened."

B. "I will need you to fill out paperwork preventing anyone from telling your spouse."

C. "Why don't you want me to tell your spouse?"

D. "Is there someone else you would like listed as an appropriate person with whom we can discuss your care?"

Rationale:

Correct answer: D

Patients have the right to decide what information regarding their condition is shared with whom. It is the responsibility of the nurse to obtain this information from the patient and document it in the medical record so others following in care will know as well. Clarifying the patient statement and determining who the patient wants involved is the best response.

A is incorrect because the nurse does not have to inform the spouse if the patient requests it.

B is incorrect because it does not facilitate open communication or clarify the patient's wishes. Documentation is not more important than clarifying the patient's wishes.

C is incorrect because it does not facilitate open communication, although it is important to know why the patient does not want their spouse informed.

18. The nurse is caring for a 72-year-old patient who has a history of a left-sided stroke. The patient uses a cane while walking. Which is the best way for the nurse to assess the strength of their lower extremities?

    A. Have the patient push with their feet against the nurse's hands

    B. Observe the patient walking in the hall

    C. Notify the physical therapy department and request an assessment

    D. Assist the patient to the bathroom

Rationale:

Correct answer: D

Patients who have experienced a stroke often have residual weakness on the affected side and use assistive devices to help with mobility. Using the cane and assisting the patient to the bathroom is the best way for the nurse to assess the patient's lower extremity strength. The nurse can assist the patient to the bathroom, and therefore, eliminate the risk for a fall.

A is incorrect because testing pedal strength only provides assessment data about the lower legs, not the full lower extremities.

B is incorrect because observing the patient walking in the hall does not give an accurate assessment of lower extremity strength and could put the patient at risk for a fall.

C is incorrect because although notifying physical therapy is an appropriate intervention, it is not the correct way for the nurse to assess the patient's lower extremity strength. This is also "passing the buck" because it is not an answer that focuses on the nurse-client interaction.

19. A patient has a urinary catheter ordered due to urinary retention. The patient should be placed in the dorsal recumbent position for the catheter insertion, but the patient states they have back pain and cannot assume that position. What is the most appropriate action the nurse should take?

    A. Place the patient in the dorsal recumbent position
    B. Place the patient on their side
    C. Place the patient in a prone position
    D. Notify the healthcare provider for an alternate order

Rationale:

Correct answer: Correct answer: B

Sterile procedure is critical when placing a urinary catheter. If the patient is unable to lie in the dorsal recumbent position for the procedure, another position such as side-lying should be used as long as the procedure can be completed in a sterile manner. Patient comfort is important as is maintaining sterile protocol during urinary catheter placement.

A is incorrect because placing the patient in a position that is painful for them puts sterile protocol at risk as well as patient comfort.

C is incorrect because prone is lying face down which is not conducive to urinary catheter placement.

D is incorrect because if the patient is experiencing urinary retention there is no alternative to the urinary catheter.

20. The nurse is caring for the Jackson-Pratt (JP) wound drain of a patient who had abdominal surgery the prior day. When cleaning the site, which technique does the nurse use?

    A. Cleaning from directly around the tube outward using a circular motion
    B. Removing the drain before cleaning the site
    C. Use alcohol to briskly wipe the site
    D. Wearing sterile gloves and a mask

Rationale:

Correct answer: A

A wound drain should be cleaned from the drain site outward using a circular motion. This will prevent contamination from the skin and a wound infection.

B is incorrect because removal of the drain is not necessary to clean the site. The drain should never be removed without a healthcare provider order.

C is incorrect because alcohol should never be used to clean a wound due to potential irritation of the site.

D is incorrect because a mask is not necessary.

- Remember: a Jackson-Pratt (JP) drain is a closed-drainage system used to prevent fluid from collecting in a wound. This reduces infection risk and allows for accurate measurement of drainage. The amount of fluid in the drain should decrease over time, as the wound heals.

21. A 64-year-old patient visits the clinic with an open wound on their foot. Which of the following strategies by the nurse is most appropriate to evaluate the patient's ability to change their dressing at home?

    A. Observe the patient changing their dressing
    B. Have the patient write down the steps of the dressing change for reference
    C. Write instructions for the patient for reference
    D. Observe the patient changing a dressing on a simulated wound model

Rationale:

Correct answer: A

Observing the patient changing the dressing will help the nurse evaluate the patient's ability.

B is incorrect because it may evaluate the patient's understanding of the steps of the dressing change, but it does not evaluate ability to implement those steps.

C is incorrect because providing instructions does not evaluate ability.

D is incorrect because performing the dressing change on a model may be helpful, but it does not evaluate ability of the patient to perform the dressing change on their own wound.

22. The nurse in the long-term care facility is assessing patients. Which of the following does the nurse identify as being at highest risk for developing decubitus ulcers?

    A. 76-year-old malnourished patient on bed rest

15

B. Obese patient who is wheelchair-bound and quit smoking one year ago

C. Incontinent patient having frequent loose stools, on a high-protein diet

D. 75-year-old patient with diabetes who is ambulatory

Rationale:

Correct answer: A

Malnourished patients are more likely to have increased bony prominences, which are susceptible to decubitus ulcers and wounds from constant pressure. Malnourishment also contributes to decreased protein levels, which are paramount in maintaining fluid status and wound healing.

B is incorrect because although obesity does contribute to risk for decubitus ulcers, this patient is not at the highest risk. Smoking is a risk factor for reduced blood flow and poor wound healing, but one year after quitting, this is not a current risk factor for decubitus ulcer.

C is incorrect because although incontinence and diarrhea increase risk for decubitus ulcers, this patient is not at the highest risk. A high–protein diet does not contribute to the development of pressure ulcers.

D is incorrect because although diabetes does contribute to the risk for decubitus ulcers, this patient is ambulatory and not at highest risk.

- Remember, risk factors for decubitus ulcers include:
    - Age: older adults have more fragile skin which regenerates less rapidly
    - Lack of sensory perception (such as spinal cord injury)
    - Excessive moisture or dryness
    - Medical conditions affecting blood flow: diabetes, peripheral vascular disease, lupus erythematosus
    - Smoking (reduces blood flow)
    - Limited alertness
    - Muscle spasms

23. The nurse is teaching a patient with newly diagnosed diabetes type 1 how to prepare an insulin syringe with 30 units of U-100 NPH insulin to self-administer. The first priority for the patient is to:

    A. Select the appropriate injection site

    B. Assess the site chosen for injection

C. Check the insulin syringe to verify correct dose has been drawn up

D. Clean the site chosen for injection with an alcohol swab

Rationale:

Correct answer: C

When a nurse teaches a patient how to prepare insulin for injection, the first priority for the patient is validating accuracy of the dose. The proper steps in order are validate dosage, select site, assess site, clean site, and inject insulin.

A is incorrect because the injection site is chosen after validating the dose.

B is incorrect because assessing the injection site is done after validating the dose and selecting the site.

D is incorrect because cleaning the site is done after validating the dose, selecting the site, and assessing the site.

24. The nurse cares for a client with an ankle splint. Which of the following assessment findings is abnormal and requires adjustment of the splint?

   A. Palpable pedal pulses
   B. Capillary refill 2 seconds in the toes
   C. The client complains of pain after the splint is applied
   D. The padding does not extend beyond the elastic bandage

Rationale:

Correct answer: D

This splint has been inappropriately placed. The padding should extend beyond the elastic bandage. The excess padding should be folded over the splint edges to form a smooth, soft border. If the elastic bandage is applied directly to the skin or if inadequate padding is used, skin breakdown can result.

A is incorrect because palpable pedal pulses is a normal finding.

B is incorrect because brisk capillary refill is a normal finding.

C is incorrect because some pain may be expected. This is a potential concern, and this finding should be investigated, but it is not as great of a physical concern as answer D, which is an actual problem.

25. The nurse is developing the discharge education plan for a patient admitted for myocardial infarction (MI). Which of the following patient statements indicates the patient is ready to follow the care plan?

A. "I don't believe I had a heart attack."

B. "I go for walks 2 or 3 times a week, usually."

C. "I will have to tell my spouse that we may not be able to have sex for a while."

D. "My job requires me to travel, so it's difficult to eat right.

Rationale:

Correct answer: C

C is a true statement. After a myocardial infarction, the heart is not healthy for vigorous exercise or sexual activity. Many doctors tell their patients not to resume sexual intercourse until the patient can climb two flights of stairs without chest pain. Other doctors will request an exercise EKG before clearing the patient for sexual activity. This statement indicates an understanding of the discharge instructions.

A is incorrect because this indicates the patient is in denial. According to Kubler-Ross, denial is the first step in the grief process after a serious life-threatening experience, such as a heart attack. The five stages are: denial, anger, bargaining, depression, and acceptance. This patient isn't likely to follow the discharge plan of care if they are still in denial.

B is incorrect because it indicates the patient may believe that walking 2-3 times a week is sufficient exercise. This statement is not dangerous for the client but it does not indicate a willingness to make lifestyle changes.

D is incorrect because the patient is resistant due to the nature of their job, so they are unlikely to be willing to make lifestyle changes.

26. The nurse is preparing to teach a 42-year-old patient with new-onset diabetes type 2 about lifestyle modifications. Which of the following characteristics demonstrate patient's readiness to learn?

    A. Moderate anxiety about administering self-injections

    B. High self-efficacy regarding assessment of the injection site

    C. Contemplating change related to the need for frequent blood glucose self-monitoring

    D. Laughing about the diagnosis, the patient states, "It seems like our bodies fall apart as we get older!"

Rationale:

Correct answer: B

Self-efficacy is important when it comes to the teaching-learning process. If a patient has high self-efficacy, they are ready to take on the problem or new diagnosis and learn everything they can in order to manage/relieve it.

A is incorrect because anxiety will only interfere with the teaching-learning process.

C is incorrect because contemplation of change means the patient has not decided if they are willing to make changes, which will not enhance teaching-learning.

D is incorrect because laughing about a health problem is a defense mechanism and the patient probably hasn't come to terms with it yet. This is a barrier to teaching-learning.

27. The nurse is teaching a 68-year-old patient recently diagnosed with osteoporosis about how to prevent fractures. Which of the following statements indicates the patient understands the instructions?

    A. "I am so glad I can still attend my dance aerobics class, as usual."
    B. "Frequent exercise will help me lose weight."
    C. I am excited to learn yoga and Pilates, with modifications for osteoporosis."
    D. "I understand I won't be able to use my elliptical machine anymore, but maybe I can start running outside when the weather is nice."

Rationale:

Correct answer: C

Osteoporosis is a condition of bone loss through decreased calcium levels as adults age. This puts patients at an increased risk for fractures. Weight-bearing and stretching exercises, including yoga and Pilates, are beneficial in osteoporosis because they can strengthen muscles and joints, and help prevent further bone loss. Estrogen replacement and calcium can additionally prevent further bone loss.

A is incorrect because dance aerobics is a high-impact activity, which increases the risk for fracture. The patient will not be able to attend their class "as usual." This would only be an acceptable exercise activity if they follow low-impact recommendations or takes a low-impact dance aerobics class. (Other examples of high-impact activities are running, jumping rope, and tennis.)

B is incorrect because, although it may be a true statement, it is not the best answer choice related to prevention of fractures.

D is incorrect because running is a high-impact activity, which strengthens muscles but does not protect bones from fracture. Elliptical use is an acceptable form of exercise for a patient with osteoporosis, as it is a low-impact option.

- Other appropriate forms of exercise for patients with osteoporosis include:
  - Stair-climbing machine
  - Fast walking on a treadmill or outside
  - Lifting weights
  - Using elastic-exercise bands
  - Swimming

28. The nurse is performing dietary teaching for a patient who experienced a myocardial infarction. Which meal choice by the patient indicates the patient understands the dietary teaching? (low-fat, low sodium)

    A. 3 oz. baked fish, baked potato with sour cream, ½ cup canned green beans, and milk
    B. 3 oz. fried salmon, steamed asparagus, garlic bread, and tea
    C. Ham sandwich, fruit salad, baked potato chips, and coffee
    D. 3 oz. roasted turkey, mashed sweet potato, ½ cup salad with light Italian dressing, and water

Rationale:

Correct answer: D

This dietary choice is low in fat and sodium and is the best choice, indicating the patient understood the dietary education. A heart-healthy diet should contain multiple servings of fruits, vegetables, and whole grains. Fat and sodium should be limited.

A is incorrect because sour cream is high in fat and canned vegetables are high in sodium.

B is incorrect because fried foods are high in fat and garlic bread is high in sodium.

C is incorrect because ham is high in fat and sodium. Although baked chips contain less fat than regular chips, they still are high in sodium.

- Examples of high-fat foods that should be avoided include red meat, fried foods, cheese, and baked goods.
- Examples of high-sodium foods that should be limited include canned products, freezer meals, smoked products, sandwich meats, and carbonated beverages.

29. The nurse supervises the nursing team caring for a patient receiving continuous enteral feeding via gastrostomy tube. The nurse will intervene when which of the following is observed?

    A. The nursing assistant completes the bed bath and then reconnects the enteral feeding with the head of the patient's bed elevated.

B. The LPN/LVN cleans around the gastrostomy tube insertion site and then applies a clean dressing.

C. The LPN verifies the patient's identity by checking the patient's hospital wristband and asking the patient to state their name.

D. The nursing assistant flushes the gastrostomy tube with 20 mL sterile water after the LPN gives the medications.

Rationale:

Correct answer: D

Flushing a gastrostomy tube is not within the nursing assistant's scope of practice. Failure to delegate appropriately is negligent, and the nurse is responsible.

A is incorrect because this is an appropriate action. It is within the nursing assistant's scope of practice to reconnect an enteral feeding tube, and the head of bed should be elevated to prevent aspiration.

B is incorrect because this is good nursing practice. It is within LPN/LVN's scope of practice to change a clean gastrostomy tube dressing.

C is incorrect because this is good nursing practice. JCAHO requires at least two patient identifiers when giving medications, collecting samples, and providing treatments or procedures. Other appropriate patient identifiers may be to ask the patient their telephone number or verify they match a picture in the patient record.

30. A patient in the rehab facility reports pain to the nurse. Which of the following is the best response by the nurse?

    A. "What pain medications have been effective in the past?"
    B. "Please describe the location and intensity of the pain."
    C. "When did the pain begin?"
    D. "Let me check when your next dose of medication is due."

Rationale:

Correct answer: B

This is the most open-ended answer choice and will give the nurse the most information. Determining the location and intensity of the pain is the priority now. This will lead to a discussion about the pain, including the pain-rating scale. (Other important assessments include: "Does the pain come and go, or is it continuous?" "What triggers the pain?")

A is incorrect because it is not the first step in pain assessment. The nurse should focus on the patient in the present. Assessment of the past is not the priority. The nurse must perform a full pain assessment and conclude with the patient's report of medication history.

C is incorrect because it is a closed-ended question, which only gives the nurse one piece of information. Answer choice B will give more detail to help the nurse help the patient.

D is incorrect because the nurse must first assess the pain. Giving pain medication is not appropriate until an assessment has been made.

31. The nurse is administering celecoxib to a patient diagnosed with arthritis. Which of the following medications on the patient's medication record could cause an interaction and adverse effects?

    A. Scopolamine
    B. Furosemide
    C. Acetaminophen
    D. Ibuprofen

Rationale:

Correct answer: D

Celecoxib is an NSAID (nonsteroidal anti-inflammatory drug) belonging to the cyclooxygenase-2 (COX-2) inhibitor group. It is used to treat pain and inflammation associated with osteoarthritis, rheumatoid arthritis, and acute pain in adults. An adverse effect of the drug is bleeding, so it shouldn't be taken with other drugs that increase bleeding including other NSAIDs, such as ibuprofen.

A is incorrect because Scopolamine does not interact with celecoxib.

B is incorrect because furosemide does not interact with celecoxib.

C is incorrect because acetaminophen does not interact with celecoxib.

32. A patient diagnosed with chronic pain is prescribed therapy with a transcutaneous electrical nerve stimulation (TENS) unit. Which statement indicates the patient understands the benefit of this type of treatment is?

    A. "I'm glad this machine will reduce the pain in my hips when getting in and out of the bathtub."
    B. "Although this method of pain control will restrict my movement, it will decrease my pain."
    C. "I'm looking forward to having more control over my pain with this treatment."
    D. "I'm glad my family will be able to care for me at home now."

Rationale:

Correct answer: C

A TENS unit delivers cutaneous stimulation which can block the pain impulse from reaching the brain, thereby reducing the sensation of the pain. The patient can initiate the signal when feeling pain, thus giving the patient control over their pain. This treatment can be performed anywhere, even in the comfort of the patient's own home.

A is incorrect because the TENS machine is not safe for use in water. If the unit is submerged, it may send excessive shock to the client and cause harm.

B is incorrect because cutaneous stimulation will increase movement as it decreases pain.

D is incorrect because a main purpose of TENS therapy is for the patient to be in charge of their pain control. Although a family member may help with care, a patient in chronic pain should be encouraged to perform as much of their own care as possible. The nurse should encourage independence.

33. A patient in the cardiac unit calls the nurse to report pain shortly after an opioid was administered. The patient has been on bed rest as part of their recovery from a myocardial infarction (MI). The patient also has a duodenal ulcer and suffers from type 1 diabetes mellitus. The nurse offers therapeutic massage because it will:

    A. Decrease fluid retention in swollen legs
    B. Decrease the pain associated with duodenal ulcers
    C. Improve circulation and muscle tightness
    D. Improve healing in diabetic wounds

Rationale:

Correct answer: C

Bed rest, despite the improvement of air mattresses, can cause muscle tension and pain over time. Therapeutic massage can improve circulation as well as decrease muscle tension. It is contraindicated in patients with deep vein thrombosis (DVT) or any condition that creates blood clots that can dislodge.

A is incorrect because therapeutic massage is not generally used for edema in lower extremities. Diuretics would help relieve this finding.

B is incorrect because therapeutic massage will not relieve pain of duodenal ulcers. Appropriate medications include proton pump inhibitors such as omeprazole.

D is incorrect because therapeutic massage will not improve healing in diabetic wounds.

34. The nurse has administered 2 mg morphine intravenously for a patient reporting pain after a Billroth's surgical procedure. Before leaving the patient's room, which of the following interventions is high priority for the nurse to perform?

    A. Leave the room light on
    B. Turn off the TV to provide a quiet atmosphere
    C. Raise the bed rails
    D. Document administration of the medication

Rationale:

Correct answer: C

Morphine is an opioid medication that can cause decreased level of consciousness, dizziness, drowsiness, and physical impairment. The nurse must ensure the bed rails are raised for patient safety before leaving the patient room. Safety is the greatest priority. (In a Billroth operation, the pylorus of the stomach is removed and the proximal stomach is connected directly to the duodenum.)

A is incorrect because leaving the room light on does not provide a restful environment or provide patient safety.

B is incorrect because turning off the TV provides a restful environment, but it does not provide patient safety.

D is incorrect because documentation of medication administration is required, but it does not provide patient safety. Direct patient care and patient safety are always prioritized ahead of documentation.

35. A patient is complaining of pain following knee replacement surgery. When the nurse prepares to administer hydromorphone, which of the following assessments is highest priority to complete prior to administration of the medication?

    A. Blood pressure
    B. Level of consciousness
    C. Respiratory rate
    D. Pain rating

Rationale:

Correct answer: C

Hydromorphone is an opioid medication that can cause drowsiness, sedation, and respiratory depression. The medication should be withheld if the patient's respiratory rate is less than 12.

A is incorrect because although hydromorphone may cause hypotension, blood pressure is not the greatest priority assessment prior to administration of hydromorphone.

B is incorrect because assessing respiratory rate is the highest priority.

D is incorrect because although pain rating may be an important part of the patient assessment prior to the administration of hydromorphone, the assessment of the airway and breathing are higher physical priority than pain.

36. The nurse administered 5 mg hydrocodone PO to a patient complaining of pain. Ten minutes later the patient experiences emesis. What is the first action the nurse should perform?

    A. Notify the healthcare provider

    B. Tell the patient, "We will wait until the nausea subsides before giving you any more pain medication."

    C. Assess the emesis for the medication

    D. Administer another dose of hydrocodone

Rationale:

Correct answer: C

Any time a patient experiences emesis, the nurse needs to inspect it for color, consistency, and amount. In this situation, the recent dose of hydrocodone warrants assessing the emesis for the pill to determine whether the patient absorbed an effective dose. The next step is to contact the healthcare provider to determine if an additional dose will be given or an antiemetic prescribed.

A is incorrect because the healthcare provider should be notified after the emesis has been assessed.

B is incorrect because steps can be taken to remedy the situation and maintain patient-centered care.

D is incorrect because administering another dose puts the patient at risk for overdose. (It is possible that the medication was absorbed by the stomach before the patient vomited, or the pill moved into the duodenum.)

37. The nurse reassesses pain 30 minutes after a patient received hydrocodone. When the patient tells the nurse he is still experiencing pain, which of the following should the nurse implement?

    A. Notify the healthcare provider for additional pain medication

    B. Guided imagery

C. Administer an additional dose of hydrocodone

D. Ambulate the patient

Rationale:

Correct answer: B

Guided imagery is a method of distraction in which the patient envisions themselves in a different place experiencing something pleasant. This can be effective in decreasing pain without medication.

A is incorrect because this patient was just medicated with an opioid 30 minutes ago and it is too early for more medication. Nonpharmacological interventions should be used for relieving his pain.

C is incorrect because the nurse cannot administer another dose of medication without an order. This is an unsafe nursing action and can lead to overdose.

D is incorrect because ambulation is not effective for clients who complain of continued pain.

38. A patient has a morphine sulfate patient-controlled analgesia (PCA) pump for pain post-thoracotomy. Which of the following interventions does the nurse perform to prevent adverse effects?

   A. Teach the patient to perform deep breathing and use incentive spirometry four times daily
   B. Administer fiber supplements to prevent constipation
   C. Teach the family members that no one should press the button except the patient
   D. Tell the patient the button can only be pressed every 15 minutes

Rationale:

Correct answer: C

Morphine is an opioid analgesic that is commonly used in PCA pumps to relieve pain. A thoracotomy is a surgery performed on the lung for several purposes including removal of infected tissue or removal of cancer. PCA pumps are frequently utilized with patients post-thoracic surgery such as thoracotomy. The patient and family should be taught that the patient is the only one who can push the button that delivers the pain medication. Others can seriously misjudge the patient's level of sedation resulting in over-sedation and respiratory depression. Opiates are one of four classes of medications that cause more than 60% of serious adverse events in the U.S. (others are insulin, anticoagulants, and antibiotics).

A is incorrect because although encouraging deep breathing and use of the incentive spirometer is important post-thoracic surgery, it should be encouraged 10 times per hour, while awake.

B is incorrect because, although administration of fiber supplements can help prevent the constipation associated with opioid medications, this is not a greater priority than preventing respiratory depression.

D is incorrect because telling the patient the PCA button can only be pushed every 15 minutes will not prevent adverse effects of morphine. The PCA is designed for the patient to administer their own pain medication as often as they feel necessary. The nurse will set limits on the pump to prevent overdose. The nurse should assess the patient and the pump frequently to determine level of consciousness, pain rating, and frequency of demand.

39. The nurse on the cardiac unit is caring for a patient who is experiencing a myocardial infarction (MI). When the patient complains of chest pain, the nurse administers sublingual nitroglycerin (NTG). The nurse instructs the patient to place the tablet:

    A. On top of the tongue

    B. On the roof of the mouth

    C. On the floor of the mouth under the tongue

    D. Between the cheek and gums

Rationale:

Correct answer: C

Sublingual nitroglycerin is given to patients experiencing myocardial infarction because it dilates the coronary arteries. It is given under the tongue on the floor of the mouth to dissolve directly into the bloodstream. This medication may cause vasodilation and thus, blood pressure should be monitored. Other forms of nitroglycerin include oral extended-release capsules, transdermal patch, and intravenous drip.

A is incorrect because nitroglycerin is not administered on top of the tongue.

B is incorrect because nitroglycerin is not administered on the roof of the mouth.

D is incorrect because nitroglycerin is not administered via the buccal route.

40. The nurse cares for a patient admitted to the medical floor with a diagnosis of liver failure and a history of Raynaud's syndrome. While reviewing the medical record, which order should the nurse question?

    A. CBC, CMP, and urinalysis upon admission

    B. Acetaminophen 325 mg PO every 4 hours as needed for pain

    C. Furosemide 40 mg IV every 12 hours

    D. EKG in AM

Rationale:

Correct answer: B

Tylenol is a non-opioid analgesic that is metabolized by the liver and is contraindicated in patients who are experiencing hepatic dysfunction. Acetaminophen can exacerbate the liver failure. The nurse should contact the healthcare provider to obtain an alternate order for pain medication.

A is incorrect because CBC, CMP, and urinalysis are routine tests which may help identify the extent of the liver failure.

C is incorrect because furosemide does not pose a risk to the patient in liver failure. The furosemide may help the kidneys diurese extra fluid in the body due to the liver failure.

D is incorrect because an EKG does not pose a risk to the patient in liver failure.

41. A patient is admitted to the medical-surgical unit with a closed head injury and confusion. Which of the following interventions does the nurse implement to keep the patient safe?

    A. Leave the bed in the low position with the side rails down so the patient can go to the bathroom
    B. Restrain the patient so they don't attempt to get out of bed
    C. Admit the patient to a room close to the nurses' station
    D. Call the healthcare provider to request a sedative medication

Rationale:

Correct answer: C

Patients with closed head injuries such as concussions are commonly confused and require reorientation. Placing the patient in a room close to the nurses' station will make it possible for someone to visualize the patient at all times, decreasing the risk for falls and patient injury.

A is incorrect because leaving the side rails down makes for easy exit from the bed, putting the patient at risk for a fall.

B is incorrect because less restrictive measures to keep the patient safe should be used before placing restraints on the patient.

D is incorrect because a sedative could potentially worsen the patient's confusion and put them at risk for falls. Sedatives and opioid medications are generally contraindicated in patients with a closed head injury because these medications can mask signs of increasing intracranial pressure.

42. The nurse on the medical-surgical unit has just received a report on four patients. Which of the following patients should the nurse see first?

A. Patient who is one day post-op hysterectomy awaiting discharge

B. Patient who is scheduled for dialysis in two hours, reports chills

C. Patient calling for pain medication

D. Patient who is two days post hip replacement surgery complaining of shortness of breath

Rationale:

Correct answer: D

Any patient who is complaining of shortness of breath takes priority. The patient who has just had hip replacement surgery is at risk for blood clots and could be experiencing a pulmonary embolus (PE). The nurse needs to see this patient first to determine what is happening.

A is incorrect because the patient awaiting discharge is stable and does not take priority over the patient experiencing shortness of breath.

B is incorrect because although this patient needs assessment, this does not take priority over the patient experiencing shortness of breath. The nurse should see this patient second.

C is incorrect because pain is less of a priority than shortness of breath. The nurse should see this patient third.

Select All That Apply

43. The nurse working on the surgical unit knows the National Patient Safety Goals as established by Joint Commission include (Select all that apply):

    A. Using side rails and bed alarms for fall prevention

    B. Using the read-back procedure for verification of verbal and phone orders

    C. Memorizing all rules set forth by Joint Commission

    D. Performing medication reconciliation for complete medication lists and ensuring appropriate use throughout a patient's care

    E. Keeping patients involved in care and encouraging them to question their care

Rationale:

Correct answers: A, B, D

National Patient Safety Goals are set forth by Joint Commission and are modified yearly to correspond to healthcare needs. Some goals are consistent, including use of side rails and alarms to prevent falls, verification of verbal and phone orders, and performing medication reconciliation. Nurses need to be aware of these patient safety goals as they are modified and updated to keep patients safe and meet Joint Commission standards.

C is incorrect because memorizing Joint Commission rules is not a National Patient Safety goal, but it is important to be familiar with them and know where to find them.

E is incorrect because encouraging patients to question their care is not a National Patient Safety Goal, although keeping them involved is important.

44. A patient is admitted to the medical unit for COPD exacerbation. The nurse knows that chronic illnesses are characterized by (Select all that apply):

    A. Consistent and predictable course

    B. Permanent deviation from what is normal

    C. Stable and unstable phases

    D. Begin with acute illness but progress slowly

    E. Reversible pathologic changes

Rationale:

Correct answers: B, C

Chronic illnesses, like COPD, are characterized by permanent deviation from what is normal, irreversible pathologic changes, residual disability, need for rehabilitation, and need for long-term care.

A is incorrect because chronic illnesses do not have consistent or predictable courses.

D is incorrect because chronic illnesses do not begin with acute illness, although they do progress slowly — dependent upon how they are treated.

E is incorrect because chronic illnesses are characterized by irreversible pathologic changes.

45. The nurse on the medical-surgical floor is caring for a patient who had open cardiac bypass surgery five days ago. The patient has a surgical incision and requires a dressing change. The nurse knows the way to prevent infection of the incision is (Select all that apply):

    A. Using hand sanitizer every time healthcare personnel enter or leave the room

    B. Administering antibiotics

    C. Wearing gloves and a mask when changing the surgical dressing

D. Changing the surgical dressing regularly

E. Preventing visitors from entering the room

Rationale:

Correct answers: C, D

Hand hygiene is the number one way to prevent infection in surgical incisions. However, the best way to prevent spread of microorganisms is to wash thoroughly with soap and water. Alcohol-based hand sanitizer is not an appropriate substitution <u>every</u> time. Wearing gloves and a mask when changing the surgical dressing is another way to prevent infection of the site. Regular dressing changes will also prevent infection.

B is incorrect because routine use of antibiotics can lead to drug resistance in microorganisms. Prophylactic antibiotics are used carefully in surgical patients.

E is incorrect because preventing visitors will not prevent infection of the surgical site but teaching visitors about proper handwashing is a good nursing implementation.

46. The nurse is assisting a patient with ambulation when the patient reports feeling dizzy. Which of the following are appropriate actions by the nurse for patient safety? (Select all that apply):

A. Stay with the patient and call for help

B. Tell the patient to lean against the wall while the nurse gets a wheelchair

C. Have the patient sit down on the floor

D. Assist the patient to the floor if they start to fall

E. Ambulate the patient back to their room and administer an antiemetic

Rationale:

Correct answers: A, D

Patient falls are common for causing patient injuries. Calling for help while staying with the patient and assisting a patient to the floor if they start to fall are both appropriate ways to prevent patient injury.

B is incorrect because having the patient lean against the wall increases the risk for injury. The nurse should not leave the patient alone.

C is incorrect because having the patient sit down on the floor is inappropriate and unsanitary.

E is incorrect because the patient should not be made to continue to walk if dizzy, and an antiemetic is not necessarily indicated for dizziness.

47. The nurse is caring for a 65-year-old patient admitted for peritonitis. The nurse knows that which of the following can influence this patient's health beliefs and health practices? (Select all that apply):

    A. Genetic background
    B. Emotional factors
    C. Family practices
    D. Financial status
    E. Developmental stage

Rationale:

Correct answers: B, C, D, E

Many factors influence a patient's health beliefs and health practices. These factors include emotional factors, family practices, financial status, and developmental stage. All of these factors have an impact on how the patient will deal with the current illness.

A is incorrect because genetic background has no influence on health practices or health beliefs.

48. A 44-year-old patient is admitted to the cardiac unit with chest pain. Which of the following are the external factors that influence this patient's illness behavior? (Select all that apply):

    A. Perception of illness
    B. Cultural background
    C. Social group
    D. Access to healthcare
    E. Chronic illness

Rationale:

Correct answers: B, C, D

Illness behavior is influenced by both internal and external factors. External factors include cultural background, social group, and access to healthcare.

A is incorrect because patient perception of illness is an internal factor influencing illness behavior.

E is incorrect because chronic (and acute) illness is an internal factor influencing illness behavior.

49. A new mother has expressed interest in breastfeeding her infant. Which of the following would be effective as provided by the nurse? (Select all that apply):

    A. Educate the new mother when she has visitors

B. Teach at times when the infant is hungry

C. Teach when the infant is crying

D. Teach the patient and the spouse if approved by the patient

E. Ask the new mother about how she feels as a new mom and about breastfeeding when teaching is completed

Rationale:

Correct answers: B, D

Teaching is best performed when patients are ready and open to learning. Family members of adult patients can be taught as well, with the patient's approval. Breastfeeding instruction can be challenging, so the patient should be rested and the baby should be hungry but not crying.

A is incorrect because, in order to protect the patient's privacy, breastfeeding instruction should be performed when there are not visitors in the room.

C is incorrect because teaching breastfeeding is difficult and frustrating when the baby is crying.

E is incorrect because asking about the patient's feelings and beliefs regarding breastfeeding is best done at the beginning of the session.

50. The nurse is caring for four patients on the medical-surgical unit. Which of the following tasks can the nurse delegate to the unlicensed assistive personnel (UAP)? (Select all that apply):

A. Start an IV in the patient complaining of pain

B. Ambulate the patient who is two days post-op hysterectomy

C. Help a patient ambulate initially after hip replacement

D. Take vital signs on the patient receiving an IV antibiotic

E. Provide a patient with discharge instruction

Rationale:

Correct answers: B, D

Unlicensed assistive personnel (UAP) have limited training and education to assist with patient care. Their duties consist of tasks including taking vital signs, bathing, ambulating, turning, and assisting with activities of daily living for stable patients. The UAP can ambulate the two-day post-op patient and take vital signs on the patient receiving an IV antibiotic.

A is incorrect because UAPs cannot start IVs.

C is incorrect because UAPs cannot ambulate a patient who has not been assessed for ability to ambulate after surgery.

E is incorrect because UAPs cannot provide discharge instructions or other forms of patient education.

CHAPTER 2:

NCLEX-RN – FUNDAMENTALS: SKILLS & PROCEDURES

Multiple Choice

1. The nurse on the medical-surgical unit has just received a report on a new patient being admitted from the emergency room. The patient has an umbilical hernia with intestinal obstruction and is going to the OR in 4 hours for herniorrhaphy. The nurse knows the best time to prepare the room for the patient is:

    A. Once the patient arrives
    B. After the patient arrives
    C. Before the patient arrives
    D. The room is already prepared

Rationale:

Correct answer: C

The room should be prepared before the patient arrives. This allows the nurse to start the admission assessment upon arrival. Personalized care can begin immediately if the room is set up with all the needed equipment to care for the patient. If an emergency arises, a prepared room will prevent delay of intervention. Patient-centered care includes introducing yourself, delivering immediate care as needed, and providing education on the room, emergency procedures, and expected outcomes.

A is incorrect because once the patient arrives, the admission assessment should begin.

B is incorrect because if the room is not ready when the patient arrives, the assessment will be delayed and the nurse may not be prepared in the case of an emergency.

D is incorrect because hospital rooms are not already prepared for specific needs of individual patients. Additional supplies and equipment needed to properly care for this patient include a truss-pad, which provides support for the herniated area until it can be surgically corrected.

2. The nurse is preparing a patient for a scheduled procedure after the healthcare provider obtained written consent and has left the patient's room. The nurse knows if the patient understands the teaching, the patient will be able to:

   A. Tell the nurse why the procedure is going to be done
   B. Ambulate to the procedure room
   C. Use less pain medication after the procedure
   D. Be discharged as scheduled

Rationale:

Correct answer: A

The nurse is responsible for reinforcing teaching about procedures and clarifying patient concerns. Each patient should be educated regarding the purpose of procedures and how they are performed. Helping the patient understand the treatment plan gives them a better sense of control over their treatment and reduces anxiety.

B is incorrect because ambulation to the procedure room does not demonstrate understanding of teaching regarding a procedure.

C is incorrect because using less pain medication is not determined by patient education regarding a procedure.

D is incorrect because discharge scheduling is not taught when educating a patient about a procedure.

3. A patient about to be transferred to the medical-surgical unit from the intensive care unit (ICU) experiences deterioration in status. What is the first intervention the ICU nurse should implement?

   A. Initiate CPR and call for a code blue
   B. Notify the healthcare provider immediately
   C. Call the medical-surgical unit to inform them there will be a delay in the transfer
   D. Complete an incident report

Rationale:

Correct answer: B

Deterioration in patient status is an unexpected outcome that can delay transfer to a lower level of care. Stabilizing the patient and calling the healthcare provider are the priorities.

A is incorrect because CPR and code blue do not necessarily need to be initiated until further assessment information is obtained. "Deterioration" is vague and does not specifically indicate pulselessness, cardiac arrest, or asystole.

C is incorrect because notifying the accepting unit is not the priority. The nurse should focus on the patient.

D is incorrect because documenting the incident report is not priority. If an incident report is needed, it should be completed by the RN after the patient has been stabilized.

4. The nurse is preparing to discharge a 53-year-old patient from the cardiac unit after myocardial infarction (MI). The patient has a history of type 1 diabetes and osteoporosis. The patient is ready for discharge and understands aftercare when:

   A. The patient is given the discharge packet
   B. The patient asks the nurse how they are supposed to prevent falls in the home
   C. The patient tells the nurse how they plan to increase their activity and make changes to their diet
   D. The patient lists the medications they will be taking

Rationale:

Correct answer: C

The discharge process is multifaceted and can be very confusing to patients. It is essential to ensure the patient understands discharge instructions in order to prevent complications and unnecessary readmissions. The nurse must educate the patient regarding medications, activity level, dietary changes, and how to care for any procedural sites as applicable.

A is incorrect because handing the patient their discharge instruction packet does not ensure the patient understands the material. The nurse should not assume the patient will read and comprehend the information. Direct, face-to-face teaching is the best method for patient education.

B is incorrect because asking about fall prevention does not indicate an understanding of discharge instructions. This statement indicates a need for more teaching.

D is incorrect because although the patient needs to know what medications they will be taking, they also need to be able to tell the nurse why the medications are needed, when to take them, and when to notify the healthcare provider.

5. A patient in the recovery room is experiencing pain despite administration of analgesia by the nurse. Which of the following statements by the nurse is an example of therapeutic communication?

A. "I will notify the healthcare provider that you are still experiencing pain and see if we can get you some relief."

B. "This pain is a problem. What do you want me to do?"

C. "Your healthcare provider commonly under-medicates patients for pain."

D. "The pain should subside once the medication has had a chance to take full effect."

Rationale:

Correct answer: A

Therapeutic communication regarding pain should be goal-directed. In this example, the goal is better management of pain.

B is incorrect because it prevents the nurse from using critical thinking to solve the problem and is not therapeutic. The nurse should remain in charge of the patient's care and not transfer the authority to the patient. The patient should not be expected to make the nursing judgment about what should be done regarding unrelieved pain.

C is incorrect because it places blame on the healthcare provider and is not therapeutic.

D is incorrect because this is dismissive. There is not enough information in the question (what pain medication was administered, what route was used, how long ago was it given) for the nurse to make the assumption that the medication has not yet taken full effect. Unrelieved pain can be a sign of a complication and should be addressed by the nurse.

6. The nurse is preparing to educate a patient regarding administration of enoxaparin injections. Which of the following questions would be most appropriate for the nurse to ask the patient?

   A. "Are you able to use a computer?"
   B. "Is your spouse here yet?"
   C. "Are you ready to give yourself an injection?"
   D. "What is your preferred way of learning?"

Rationale:

Correct answer: D

Patient education is very important for patients to understand how injections are performed in order to prevent errors and complications. Everyone has different learning styles, so the nurse must identify how the patient learns best in order to provide appropriate patient education.

A is incorrect because use of a computer is unrelated to learning how to self-inject enoxaparin.

Patients should not be encouraged to use the internet to learn about medication administration, as the nurse can't be sure that the information they find will be accurate. The nurse is responsible for the teaching.

B is incorrect because the spouse does not necessarily need to be present for teaching to begin. Assessing the patient's learning style should be done first. The nurse must focus on teaching the patient. Education should not be delayed because a family member is not present. It is important to teach those who will be assisting in the patient's care at home, but that can be done later.

C is incorrect because it is closed-ended and is inappropriate to ask until after the patient has been educated about enoxaparin and how to safely administer this drug. The nurse may administer the injection first and then assess readiness for self-injection at the next scheduled dose.

7. The emergency room nurse is caring for a patient who has become belligerent and is yelling at the staff. Which of the following interventions by the nurse is the most appropriate for this patient?

   A. Speak clearly and louder than the patient to prevent having to repeat what the nurse has said.
   B. Stand near the door of the room and stay calm.
   C. Have other members of the healthcare team enter the room to demonstrate ability to gain control of the situation.
   D. Ask the patient about what they do at home when they feel like this.

Rationale:

Correct answer: B

Patients who are belligerent are unpredictable and may be a risk to themselves or others. Standing near the door prevents the patient from blocking the exit and allows for a rapid exit by the nurse, if necessary. The nurse should attempt to de-escalate the situation emotionally by staying calm and composed. Listen to what the patient is saying and explain that you understand that they are upset. Often the cause of anger and belligerence is fear.

A is incorrect because simply speaking louder may make the patient feel threatened and worsen the belligerence. The nurse should be compassionate and direct, make the patient feel heard, and attempt to diminish what might be causing their fear.

C is incorrect because bringing more team members in the room may be perceived by the patient as threatening and can worsen the situation.

D is incorrect because the nurse should not ask this type of question to the belligerent patient. The nurse should validate that the patient is upset and offer measures to help them calm down. It is important not to make promises that can't be fulfilled.

8. The nurse has administered dilaudid to a patient experiencing pain. When reassessing the patient's pain, the nurse discovers the patient's respirations have decreased from 22 to 8, and the patient is snoring. When documenting the occasion, which of the following statements is best?

   A. Too much dilaudid was administered; monitoring patient frequently and appears stable, family at bedside informed of the situation

   B. Incident report completed due to patient receiving too much dilaudid and experienced drop in respirations; resting quietly and charge nurse notified

   C. Dilaudid 1 mg IV push. Vitals afterward: respirations 8, blood pressure 102/72, pulse 68. Monitoring patient every 15 minutes and healthcare provider notified. See graphic for additional vital signs.

   D. Difficult to arouse after dilaudid administered; snoring respirations noted, vital signs stable, oxygen ready for administration, healthcare provider notified.

Rationale:

Correct answer: C

Documentation should be objective, giving an explanation of exactly what occurred including dosage, route, vital signs, patient status, what the nurse is doing to help the patient, and notification of the healthcare provider.

A is incorrect because it is vague documentation and does not accurately depict what occurred. The nurse should not document subjective findings such as the nurse's personal opinion that "too much" was given or how the patient "appears." This documentation does not give enough objective information such as the dose given and the actual vital signs measured.

B is incorrect because documentation of an incident report being completed should never be included in a patient's chart. The words "too much dilaudid" are the nurse's subjective opinion. It is appropriate to notify the charge nurse, but the healthcare provider who ordered the dilaudid should be notified, too.

D is incorrect because it does not state the dose given and the words "vital signs stable" are the nurse's subjective opinion.

9. The nurse is preparing to measure vital signs on a patient. When measuring respirations, which of the following is the best method?

   A. Tell the patient respirations are going to be counted

   B. Place the patient on a cardiac monitor for respiration rate

   C. Instruct the patient to take a deep breath every 4 or 5 seconds

D. Count respirations while holding the patient's wrist

Rationale:

Correct answer: D

Count the patient's respirations while holding the patient's wrist as if measuring radial pulse. This will distract the patient and help them breathe normally. This method will get the most accurate measurement for respirations. Normal adult respiratory rate is 12-2- breaths per minute. The thorax of the adult patient should rise and fall with each breath (costal breathing) with expiration lasting slightly longer than inspiration. Factors that can affect breathing include pain, fever, anxiety, drugs, and disease.

A is incorrect because telling the patient the respirations will be counted may alter their breathing.

B is incorrect because cardiac monitors are not consistently accurate in counting respirations. The nurse should rely on personal physical assessment over equipment.

C is incorrect because telling the patient to breathe at certain intervals will alter their normal breathing pattern and the nurse will not get an accurate respiration rate.

10. The unlicensed assistive personnel (UAP) has just taken vital signs on a 75-year-old patient and tells the nurse the pulse is 48 bpm. What is the best response by the nurse?

   A. "I will notify the healthcare provider immediately."
   B. "Recheck the pulse for a full minute to make sure it is accurate."
   C. "Call for a rapid response while I recheck the pulse."
   D. "Go ahead and document it in the patient's chart."

Rationale:

Correct answer: B

Unlicensed assistive personnel (UAP) are sometimes trained to check a pulse for 15 seconds and multiply by 4 (or for 30 seconds and multiply by 2 in order) to obtain a pulse rate. It is best to count the pulse for a full minute, especially in patients who have irregular heart rates. The nurse should ask the UAP to recheck the pulse.

A is incorrect because the pulse needs to be verified and the patient assessed by the nurse before the healthcare provider is unnecessarily notified.

C is incorrect because the nurse should assess the patient before calling for a rapid response. If the patient is asymptomatic, has recently received a beta-blocker, or tends to run bradycardic, a rapid response may not need to be called.

D is incorrect because the nurse should prioritize direct personal assessment of the patient with an abnormally low pulse ahead of documentation.

11. The nurse is performing a neurologic assessment on a patient admitted for possible stroke. Which of the following techniques will ensure an accurate assessment?

    A. Perform testing rapidly so stroke treatment is not delayed
    B. Administer an anxiolytic before the assessment
    C. Compare the exam from one side of the body to the other
    D. Place the patient in the supine position

Rationale:

Correct answer: C

Comparing the physical assessment findings on both sides of the body is imperative when stroke is suspected. This will ensure the affected and unaffected sides are covered during the assessment.

A is incorrect because rapid assessment risks an incomplete assessment and omission of unaffected or affected areas. While thrombolytic medications should be started quickly if stroke is confirmed, it is most important for the nurse not to rush, but to obtain an accurate and thorough neurological exam.

B is incorrect because administration of an anxiolytic medication may affect the neurologic abilities of the patient.

D is incorrect because the patient does not need to be supine for neurologic assessment.

12. The nurse has just completed a respiratory assessment on a patient and noted high-pitched musical sounds. These sounds would be documented as:

    A. Normal vesicular sounds
    B. Rhonchi
    C. Crackles
    D. Wheezes

Rationale:

Correct answer: D

Wheezes are usually high-pitched, squeaky, and musical in nature. Wheezes indicate a narrowing of the airways and are not an expected finding in the respiratory assessment.

A is incorrect because vesicular sounds are soft, breezy, and low-pitched. Vesicular sounds are common and expected.

B is incorrect because rhonchi are similar to blowing air through a fluid with a straw, or coarse, rattling vibrations heard on expiration.

C is incorrect because crackles are similar to crushing cellophane or tearing Velcro.

13. The nurse is performing the respiratory assessment on a 64-year-old patient and believes crackles are heard. Which of the following should the nurse do to confirm the findings?

    A. Ask the patient if they have had crackles before
    B. Have the patient breathe through their nose
    C. Have the patient breathe deeper when auscultating the bases of the lungs
    D. Check the patient's medical record to see if crackles were auscultated previously

Rationale:

Correct answer: C

Encouraging deep breathing while auscultating lung bases will assist in fully assessing all lung sounds and confirm the presence of crackles.

A is incorrect because patients generally do not auscultate their own lung sounds. The patient may not know whether crackles have been heard before. The nurse should rely on personal observation and assessment, rather than relying on the patient's recall of their history.

B is incorrect because breathing through the nose will not change how the lung sounds are heard and may even prevent deep breathing needed for auscultating lung sounds.

D is incorrect because the nurse should confirm what was heard before referring to previous documentation.

14. A patient is admitted with *Clostridium difficile* infection. The nurse on the medical unit knows the best way to prevent transmission of this highly contagious pathogen includes:

    A. Wearing a mask when caring for the patient
    B. Using soap and water for hand hygiene
    C. Using hand sanitizer when entering and leaving the patient's room
    D. Maintaining droplet precautions

Rationale:

Correct answer: B

C. difficile is an infection that causes chronic diarrhea and is easily spread from person to person. The patient must be placed on contact precautions and soap and water used for hand hygiene.

A is incorrect because *C. difficile* is not airborne.

C is incorrect because hand sanitizer does not effectively remove *C. difficile* spores from the hands.

D is incorrect because C. difficile does not require droplet precautions.

15. The nurse is preparing to perform a sterile dressing change on a patient with an abdominal wound. When setting up the sterile field which of the following actions would compromise the sterile field?

    A.   Using clean gloves to set up the supplies on the sterile field and then changing into sterile gloves
    B.   Dropping the sterile supplies on the field and maintaining the 1-inch border
    C.   Picking up the first sterile glove by the inside of the cuff
    D.   Keeping the sterile gloved hands at chest level

Rationale:

Correct answer: A

Sterile gloves should be used when arranging sterile supplies on the sterile field. All supplies are opened then dropped onto the sterile field, then sterile gloves put on, and supplies arranged maintaining a 1-inch border around the field.

B is incorrect because it is correct technique for sterile supplies.

C is incorrect because it is correct technique for donning sterile gloves.

D is incorrect because sterile gloved hands should be kept at or above the level of the waist to maintain sterility.

16. A patient is in the medical-surgical unit after laparotomy. Two hours after admission, the nurse attempts to reposition the patient in bed and the patient refuses. Which of the following should be assessed by the nurse first?

    A.   Oxygen saturation
    B.   Pain level
    C.   Level of consciousness
    D.   Patient lifting equipment available

Rationale:

Correct answer: B

A laparotomy is a surgical incision made in the abdomen. The patient's pain level may be elevated, leading to increased pain when moving or being repositioned. The nurse should assess for pain and provide pain medication as needed before attempting to reposition again.

A is incorrect because refusal to be repositioned is not a sign of hypoxia. Assessment findings that indicate oxygen deprivation include restlessness, agitation, confusion, drowsiness, altered level of consciousness, and disorientation.

C is incorrect because refusal to cooperate with repositioning is likely a sign of pain. Decreased level of consciousness presents as drowsiness and disorientation, but not non-compliance or refusal of care.

D is incorrect because the availability of patient lifting equipment would not affect the patient's willingness to be repositioned. Determining if patient lifting equipment is available does not address the patient's resistance to care.

17. The nurse attempts to get a patient up to a chair after several days on bed rest. When placed upright, the patient becomes dizzy and nauseated. The nurse realizes that the patient is experiencing:

   A. Rebound hypertension
   B. Dysfunctional proprioception
   C. Dehydration and fluid-volume deficit
   D. Orthostatic hypotension

Rationale:

Correct answer: D

Orthostatic hypotension occurs when the blood pressure drops in response to a patient changing positions from lying supine to being seated upright and standing. It can indicate several things including dehydration, fever, or any condition causing vasodilation.

A is incorrect because rebound hypertension occurs after prolonged bed rest.

B is incorrect because signs of dysfunctional proprioception is the inability to distinguish body position in relation to the patient's surrounding space. Symptoms include clumsiness, lack of coordination, and poor postural stability.

C is incorrect because no information is given to suggest the patient is dehydrated. Bed rest for several days can cause blood pressure to drop when changing from horizontal to vertical position, so the hypotension is likely orthostatic, not fluid-volume related.

18. The nurse suspects one of the patients has a deep vein thrombosis (DVT) after being on bed rest. What priority nursing intervention does the nurse need to implement?

    A. Test for Homans' sign
    B. Massage the leg to promote circulation
    C. Make sure the patient is calm and notify the healthcare provider
    D. Apply sequential compression devices (SCDs)

Rationale:

Correct answer: C

DVTs commonly form in patients who are subject to immobility. If a DVT is suspected, the patient should be kept calm in bed, and the healthcare provider notified immediately. The nurse will anticipate a DVT scan will be performed at the bedside, and blood-thinners will be started if the scan reveals a DVT.

A is incorrect because Homans' sign is no longer used to test for DVT. Dorsiflexing the patient's foot can actually cause a DVT to become dislodged and travel through the body.

B is incorrect because massaging the leg is contraindicated as it can break any clots loose and cause MI, PE, or stroke.

D is incorrect because SCDs are contraindicated if a clot is suspected. The compression can break clots loose and cause MI, PE, or stroke.

19. A patient has just been taught by the nurse about how to get up independently from a seated position in the chair to a standing position with their walker. Which of the following patient statements indicates the patient understood the teaching?

    A. "I will use the handgrips of the walker for leverage."
    B. "I will scoot to the back of the chair before I get up."
    C. "I will rock a few times before getting up."
    D. "I will use the chair arms to push myself up to the walker."

Rationale:

Correct answer: D

The arms of a chair are more stable for use when standing up to a walker. If the patient is not able to fully rise when attempting to stand, the fall will be back into the chair.

A is incorrect because the walker may tip over causing a fall. The patient should stabilize themselves with the chair arms instead.

B is incorrect because the patient should scoot to the front or edge of the chair.

C is incorrect because rocking is used when another person is assisting the patient to stand. This patient is practicing independently transitioning from a seated position to a standing position.

20. The nurse is preparing to assist a patient with ambulation. The patient has been experiencing left-sided weakness. Which of the following actions is most appropriate for assisting this patient with ambulation?

    A. Delegate ambulation assistance to the strongest healthcare worker
    B. Walk on the patient's left side during ambulation
    C. Have the patient hold the cane in the left hand and walk behind the patient
    D. Walk on the patient's right side

Rationale:

Correct answer: B

For the best support, the nurse should walk on the patient's left side. This allows the nurse to provide assistance with the weak side.

A is incorrect because delegating support to the strongest individual is not necessary. All healthcare workers should be adequately trained and capable of ambulating patients of differing sizes.

C is incorrect because walking behind the patient does not provide for safety. If the patient has difficulty with ambulation, they will need support on their left side. The cane should be held on the strong side of the body.

D is incorrect because walking on the patient's right side, or strong side, places the patient at risk for a fall.

21. A patient has had a back brace applied, and the nurse is teaching them how to use it properly. Which instructions should be included by the nurse for this patient?

    A. No clothing should be worn under the back brace
    B. Inspect the back brace daily for damage, rough edges, and wear
    C. Clean metal joints with a steel brush and emollient should be applied to joints every two weeks
    D. Clean the plastic of the back brace weekly with a half-strength ammonia solution

Rationale:

Correct answer: B

It is important to inspect the brace regularly as rough edges and excessive wear or damage can cause skin breakdown or lack of stability and spinal support.

A is incorrect because a cotton shirt should be worn under the brace for skin protection. Often, a back brace is worn for 23 hours each day (usually only removed for showering or bathing). If it is worn with no clothing protection underneath, this will cause skin breakdown.

C is incorrect because the joints are cleaned with pipe cleaners weekly and oiled.

D is incorrect because ammonia can be damaging to the plastic. The brace should be cleaned with mild soap and water and thoroughly dried before reapplying to the patient.

22. The nurse is in the trauma unit caring for a patient in skeletal traction. Which of the following precautions would be appropriate for this patient?

    A. Avoid placing an overhead trapeze on the bed
    B. Remove the weights when repositioning the patient
    C. Make sure the affected limb and the trunk maintain alignment
    D. Every eight hours, traction is relieved for 15 minutes

Rationale:

Correct answer: C

Skeletal traction is used to realign fractured bones. The affected limb and the trunk must be in alignment for the traction to perform proper pull.

A is incorrect because an overhead trapeze should be used for repositioning. This allows the patient some independence with changing position and can help prevent skin breakdown.

B is incorrect because it is not within the nurse's scope of practice to remove the weights in skeletal traction. This can delay healing. Skeletal traction is also very painful, so the nursing team must use extreme caution not to bump the bed or touch the weights, causing them to swing.

D is incorrect because weights are never removed from skeletal traction, as this will delay healing. Due to the extreme pain associated with traction, the nurse should be prepared to administer analgesics and anti-muscle-spasm medications. These patients are also at risk for sensory deprivation, boredom, and depression. So, it is important for the nurse to interact with the patient frequently and provide stimulation and activities to keep the patient occupied.

23. The nurse finds a patient unconscious on the floor, and the nurse suspects they have a head injury from a fall. What is the first action the nurse should perform to prevent the patient from being injured further?

    A. Perform a head-to-toe assessment
    B. Apply a cervical collar
    C. Delegate three assistants to carefully return the patient to bed
    D. Notify the healthcare provider

Rationale:

Correct answer: B

Any time a head or neck injury is suspected, a cervical collar should be applied. This is the only option that prevents further injury to the patient.

A is incorrect because an assessment will not prevent further injury to the patient.

C is incorrect because returning the patient to the bed without a C-collar can cause further damage. The nurse must apply the C-collar and immediately assess the patient before changing their position.

D is incorrect because notifying the healthcare provider will not prevent further injury to the patient. The nurse should stay with the patient and delegate another member of the nursing team to call the healthcare provider.

24. The nurse applies restraints to a patient who is trying to pull out invasive lines. Which of the following actions must the nurse perform within an hour of applying the restraints in order to meet Joint Commission standards?

    A. Educate the patient regarding restraints
    B. Notify the patient's spouse
    C. Notify the healthcare provider to assess the patient
    D. Document the application of the restraints

Rationale:

Correct answer: C

Restraints are applied to prevent a patient from harming themselves, including pulling out invasive lines such as arterial lines and central lines. A patient who has restraints applied must be seen by the healthcare provider within one hour to justify application of the restraints. This is a Joint Commission standard.

A is incorrect because explaining the restraints to the patient is not a Joint Commission standard.

B is incorrect because notifying the spouse is not a Joint Commission standard. However, if the spouse is at the bedside, the nurse should explain the use of the restraints.

D is incorrect because documenting the restraints within an hour is not a Joint Commission standard, although alternate methods and application of the restraints as well as neurovascular checks and essential needs met must be documented.

25. A patient on the oncology unit calls the nurse to report a fire coming from an electrical socket. Which of the following actions by the nurse is inappropriate?

    A. Shut off oxygen supply to the room
    B. Evacuate the patient from the room
    C. Pull the fire alarm
    D. Instruct a UAP to use the fire extinguisher and then promptly remove the patient from the room

Rationale:

Correct answer: D

The proper response to a fire is RACE: Rescue, Alert, Contain, Evacuate. The patient should be rescued before attempts are made to extinguish the fire. A fire extinguisher may cause further harm if used on an electrical fire.

A is incorrect because turning off oxygen to a room where there is a fire is an appropriate action.

B is incorrect because evacuating the patient from the room is an appropriate action.

C is incorrect because pulling the fire alarm is an appropriate action.

26. A patient is brought to the emergency department with possible cutaneous anthrax. Which precautions should the staff take?

    A. Standard
    B. Contact
    C. Respiratory
    D. Airborne

Rationale:

Correct answer: B

Anthrax is caused by gram-positive *Bacillus anthracis* and causes serious infections. It is a rare type of infection transmitted through contact with anthrax spores. Because of the mode of transmission, the patient should be placed on contact isolation as this is a cutaneous exposure. All types of anthrax have the potential, if untreated, to spread throughout the body and cause severe illness and even death.

A is incorrect standard precautions are not sufficient to prevent transmission of this type of anthrax. Standard precautions are needed for a patient admitted with anthrax inhalation, which is not spread from person to person.

C is incorrect because this is not a respiratory exposure of anthrax.

D is incorrect because this is not an airborne exposure of anthrax.

27. The nurse is caring for patients in the intensive care unit. The nurse knows bathing provided at regular intervals will:

    A. Restore pH of the skin
    B. Remove bacteria from open wounds
    C. Clean the outer layer of skin and remove dead skin cells
    D. Promote maturation of new skin cells

Rationale:

Correct answer: C

Bathing patients at regular intervals with washcloths will clean the skin and remove dead skin cells.

A is incorrect because regular bathing does not affect skin pH.

B is incorrect because, when bathing a patient, open wounds are to be covered. Irrigation or debridement (not bathing) will help remove bacteria from wounds.

D is incorrect because regular bathing may remove dead skin cells and stimulate growth of new ones, but does not promote maturation of the new skin cells.

28. The nurse in the intensive care unit is caring for an unresponsive patient with a head injury. The patient arouses with painful stimuli. Which of the following assessments performed by the nurse is the most crucial to determine safety of performing oral hygiene?

    A. Check pupil responses
    B. Evaluate the patient's Glasgow Coma Scale
    C. Assess oral cavity
    D. Assess presence of gag reflex

Rationale:

Correct answer: D

Assessing for the presence of a gag reflex will determine if the patient could aspirate fluids during oral care. Decreased or no gag reflex means high risk of aspiration.

A is incorrect because pupil response does not necessarily indicate the presence of a gag reflex and is not related to safety when performing oral care.

B is incorrect because the Glasgow Coma Scale determines level of consciousness but does not give specific information related to aspirating during oral care.

C is incorrect because although it is important to assess the oral cavity, it will not determine risk for aspiration.

29. The nurse is caring for a patient with severe partial thickness burns to the face and chest. The patient has been unable to be weaned from the ventilator since the injuries were sustained in a fire, six days ago. Which of the following implementations will the nurse perform to decrease the risk of ventilator-assisted pneumonia (VAP) in this intubated patient?

    A. Peroxide
    B. Normal saline
    C. Chlorhexidine
    D. Tap water oral rinsing

Rationale:

Correct answer: C

VAP occurs in patients who are intubated and on the ventilator for more than 24 hours. VAP can be prevented by using chlorhexidine oral solution for frequent oral care, keeping the head of the bed at least 30 degrees elevation, and frequent endotracheal suctioning.

A is incorrect because peroxide is not recommended for oral care in ventilated patients as it can cause breakdown of the mucous membranes inside the mouth.

B is incorrect because normal saline does not kill bacteria and has not been shown to prevent VAP.

D is incorrect because tap water does not prevent VAP.

30. The nurse is caring for patients on the medical-surgical unit. The nurse receives an order for hydrocolloid dressings to be used for pressure ulcers on the patient's elbow and scapula. The nurse knows the purpose of using a hydrocolloid dressing is what?

A. Hydrocolloid dressings provide an antibiotic solution for killing surface bacteria, thus promoting healing

B. Hydrocolloid dressings protect wound bases and maintain a moist environment

C. Hydrocolloid dressings can be changed frequently and not cause damage to the wound bed

D. Hydrocolloid dressings perform debriding for a clean wound environment

Rationale:

Correct answer: B

Hydrocolloid dressings are used to maintain a moist environment to protect the wound base and support growth of new tissue.

A is incorrect because hydrocolloid dressings do not provide antibiotics.

C is incorrect because hydrocolloid dressings require changing only every 3-5 days.

D is incorrect because hydrocolloids do not debride.

31. The nurse is assessing patients on the medical-surgical unit for pressure ulcer risk. Which of the following patients is at greatest risk?

A. 75-year-old patient with Alzheimer's and poor oral intake

B. 48-year-old patient with paraplegia in a wheelchair

C. 56-year-old patient with diabetes type I who is post-op day one cardiac surgery and has been diaphoretic

D. 65-year-old patient who had bladder surgery and is incontinent

Rationale:

Correct answer: C

This patient has three risk factors for development of a pressure ulcer: diabetes type I (the disease process impairs vasculature and sensation), limited mobility due to surgery, and diaphoresis (which leaves skin moist and at greater risk for tearing.)

A is incorrect because this patient has one risk factor: poor intake

B is incorrect because this patient has one risk factor: wheelchair-bound

D is incorrect because this patient has one risk factor: incontinence

32. The nurse is caring for a patient who has developed severe conjunctivitis. The patient wears contact lenses. When the nurse educates the patient regarding prevention of recurrent conjunctivitis, which statement by the patient indicates a knowledge deficit?

  A. "Any open contact lens solutions should be discarded once I get home."
  B. "Any solution that is cloudy should be discarded."
  C. "Household hand soap for handwashing is sufficient before handling contact lenses."
  D. "I'll be requesting disposable contacts so there's no risk for infection."

Rationale:

Correct answer: D

All types of contact lenses carry a risk of becoming contaminated and causing conjunctivitis. Some contact lenses are reusable, requiring proper washing in-between insertion. The patient should be taught the importance of proper handwashing when handling the contact lenses, and the importance of following all manufacturer's guidelines pertaining to the insertion and care of the contact lenses.

Conjunctivitis (also known as pinkeye) is conjunctiva inflammation. It is characterized by pink color to the sclera of the eye, due to conjunctival blood vessel hemorrhage. General symptoms include: a feeling of a foreign body in the eye, scratching or burning sensation, photophobia, and exudate from the eye. Conjunctiva can be unilateral or bilateral. The most common causes of bacterial conjunctivitis are *Strep. pneumoniae, H. influenza,* and *Staph. aureus.*

A is incorrect because it is a true statement. Any open container of contact lens solution at home may have already been contaminated with the bacteria that caused the conjunctivitis. The patient should be instructed to start with a fresh, new, unopened bottle of solution after being treated for conjunctivitis.

B is incorrect because it is a true statement; contact lens solutions should be clear. Cloudy fluid suggests contamination and should not be used.

C is incorrect because it is a true statement; proper handwashing before handling contact lenses is important to prevent contamination, and no specific soap is required. Other instructions for patients who wear contact lenses (to prevent conjunctivitis) include avoiding rubbing the eyes and do not share towels or washcloths with others.

33. A patient who wears bilateral hearing aids tells the nurse they have discomfort in the right ear. What is the first intervention the nurse should perform?

  A. Ask the patient if they understand hearing aid care

B. Assess the ears for inflammation

C. Teach the patient how to reposition hearing aids to decrease discomfort

D. Turn down the volume of the left ear hearing aid

Rationale:

Correct answer: B

The ears must be assessed by the nurse before any interventions are performed. Any irritation, inflammation, or infection must be identified. What is found during assessment determines the most appropriate intervention.

A is incorrect because although improper care of hearing aids could cause irritation, it is not the first intervention. The nurse should perform a thorough physical assessment before assuming a knowledge deficit is present.

C is incorrect because although it is appropriate to teach repositioning hearing aids, it is not the first intervention. Physical assessment must be done first.

D is incorrect because turning down the volume on the unaffected ear is inappropriate. If the nurse is going to remove the hearing aid and assess the right ear, the aid in the left ear should remain in place with the volume on so the patient can hear the nurse during the assessment process.

34. A patient in the clinic tells the nurse they are experiencing increasing pain in the right ear. What initial response by the nurse is best?

A. "Squirt a small amount of soapy water to clean your ears daily."

B. "Clean out as much earwax as you can."

C. "Put a couple of drops of mineral oil in your right ear."

D. "Can you describe the ear pain to me?"

Rationale:

Correct answer: D

The nurse's first response should be to get more information pertaining to the ear pain the patient is experiencing. Signs and symptoms to be ascertained include presence of drainage and odor, as well as quality and severity of the pain. Once all pertinent information is collected, an intervention can be performed based on the assessment.

A is incorrect because injecting soap and water is appropriate for cleaning ears, and this is not pertinent to the situation. The patient should be taught not to insert anything into the ears. Ears can be cleaned daily with a damp washcloth, cleaning only as far in as the patient can comfortably reach with one finger covered by the washcloth, applying light pressure only.

B is incorrect because not all earwax needs to be cleaned out of the ears. Earwax has protective mechanisms. If a patient needs earwax removed from the ear due to excessive buildup, the healthcare provider should be notified. Manually attempting to remove earwax from the ear can potentially rupture the tympanic membrane.

C is incorrect because patients should be taught not to insert or inject anything into the ear. The tympanic membrane must be assessed for intactness before the healthcare provider will make a determination if any solution needs to be used to irrigate the ear.

35. A patient is brought to the emergency department with sudden onset dyspnea. Which of the following symptoms would the nurse expect to find upon assessment?

    A. Respiratory rate of 26 bpm
    B. Bradycardia
    C. Clubbed fingers
    D. Regular breathing pattern

Rationale:

Correct answer: A

Dyspnea is difficulty breathing, which can be attributed to several different problems. A patient experiencing dyspnea will most likely have an increased respiratory rate or tachypnea. If the brain is not receiving enough oxygen, it will send signals to the respiratory muscles to increase rate of respiration in an attempt to meet oxygen demand. Heart rate may also increase as a compensatory mechanism in response to decreased oxygenation.

B is incorrect because the nurse would expect to assess tachycardia in a patient who is dyspneic.

C is incorrect because clubbed fingers are seen after prolonged hypoxia and chronic lung disease.

D is incorrect because a regular breathing pattern is not indicative of a problem.

36. The nurse has applied an oxygen mask to a patient experiencing dyspnea. Which of the following assessments should the nurse make, initially, to determine if the oxygen therapy is effective?

    A. Mucous membrane color
    B. Arterial blood gas
    C. Pulse oximetry
    D. Lung sounds

Rationale:

Correct answer: C

Pulse oximetry is a measurement of capillary arterial oxygen saturation. This method gives immediate feedback on the effectiveness of oxygen therapy.

A is incorrect because bluish color to mucous membranes is a late sign of hypoxia. If oxygen therapy is effective, normal color will return to the mucous membranes over time. This will not give the earliest information about the effectiveness of oxygen.

B is incorrect because obtaining an ABG takes time; this is not something the nurse can assess at the bedside. It is quicker to check the pulse oximetry reading, which should increase immediately if the amount of oxygen is appropriate for the dyspneic patient.

D is incorrect because lung sounds do not demonstrate adequacy of oxygen therapy.

37. A patient is being treated with oxygen therapy via oxygen mask with reservoir (non-rebreather). If the reservoir bag deflates, which of the following would the patient experience?

    A. Increased oxygen levels
    B. Elevated carbon dioxide levels
    C. Drying of mucous membranes
    D. Decreased respiratory rate

Rationale:

Correct answer: B

A non-rebreather oxygen mask delivers 80-100% oxygen at up to 12L per minute. This type of mask is used to prevent increased carbon dioxide levels by blocking carbon dioxide from being inhaled from the mask through special one-way valves. The reservoir should be 2/3 filled with oxygen during inspiration. If it becomes deflated, the patient will experience an increase in carbon dioxide levels.

A is incorrect because the oxygen levels would decrease if the bag deflated.

C is incorrect because deflation of the reservoir would not dry out the mucous membranes. Any type of oxygen therapy has the potential to dry out mucous membranes. Thus, the nurse should apply water-soluble lubrication to the nose and lips and provide oral care routinely. Skin should be washed and dried routinely, with lotion applied to the face to prevent drying of the skin.

D is incorrect because deflation of the reservoir would not cause a decrease in respiration rate.

38. A patient admitted for acute pneumonia has a 15-year history of chronic lung disease and is unable to clear respiratory secretions. Which of the following suctioning interventions is appropriate for this patient?

   A. Oropharyngeal
   B. Nasopharyngeal
   C. Endotracheal
   D. Tracheal

Rationale:

Correct answer: A

A patient who is unable to clear secretions would need oropharyngeal suction to remove thick mucus in large amounts. This can be done with a Yankauer or tonsillar tip suction device. The patient should be hyper-oxygenated before suctioning. The tip of the suction device should be moistened with sterile saline before insertion. Wall suction should be set at 80-120 mm Hg. Postural drainage and frequent coughing and turning are also appropriate for this patient. Percussion and vibration can additionally be performed during postural drainage to facilitate the effect of gravity drainage.

B is incorrect because nasopharyngeal suction would be inappropriate. If the nurse is able to suction via the mouth, it is often less uncomfortable than through the patient's nasal passages.

C is incorrect because endotracheal suction cannot be performed without an endotracheal tube.

D is incorrect because tracheal suction cannot be performed without a tracheal airway, such as a tracheostomy.

39. A patient is admitted to the intensive care unit after a thoracotomy procedure. The vital signs at the end of the procedure were: BP 118/72, HR 64, RR 18, SPO_2 99% and temperature 98.1°F (36.7°C). Which of the following manifestations is most concerning to the nurse after a thoracotomy?

   A. Increased mentation
   B. Feeling of euphoria
   C. Heart rate 89 and sinus rhythm with occasional premature ventricular contractions (PVCs)
   D. Lethargy

Rationale:

Correct answer: D

A thoracotomy is an incision into the pleural space of the chest used by a surgeon to gain access to major organs in the thorax. Thoracotomy incisions are extremely painful and can lead to shallow breathing, which can cause hypoxia, atelectasis, or pneumonia. Common manifestations of hypoxia include lethargy, restlessness, agitation, confusion, and anxiety. The nurse may also see tachycardia and dysrhythmias related to hypoxia.

A is incorrect because patients experiencing hypoxia will have a decreased level of consciousness.

B is incorrect because euphoria is not a sign of hypoxia and is not related to thoracotomy.

C is incorrect because tachycardia and dysrhythmias are common with hypoxia. This patient's HR has increased from 64 to 89 (likely due to the anesthesia wearing off), and this HR is still within normal limits. Occasional PVCs are not an immediate threat. These may be caused by high calcium or low potassium (neither are related to thoracotomy), adrenaline, alcohol, caffeine, and cocaine.

40. The nurse is caring for a patient with a tracheostomy whose pulse oximeter has decreased from 90% five minutes ago to 85% currently. What is the priority action by the nurse?

    A. Check for a pulse
    B. Assess blood pressure
    C. Check that the airway is patent
    D. Check oxygen supply connections

Rationale:

Correct answer: C

When oxygen saturation drops, the nurse should first assess the patency of the airway. The nurse must first determine if the airway is occluded, in order to determine how to intervene next.

A is incorrect because sudden decrease of oxygen saturation does not indicate pulse has been lost. Pulse is an assessment of circulation, but the problem here is oxygenation, so the nurse must address the airway.

B is incorrect because blood pressure is also an assessment of circulation and is not priority over airway assessment.

D is incorrect because although an interrupted oxygen supply may be the cause of the problem, the nurse must assess the patient's physical status ahead of checking equipment.

41. The ICU nurse is caring for a patient with a head injury who has decompensated. An oral endotracheal tube was recently inserted at the bedside, and the patient was placed on a ventilator. The healthcare provider left the room quickly to resuscitate another patient in a nearby room. The nurse notes the

patient has unequal breath sounds, the respiration rate is 16 breaths per minute, and the SPO_2 is 97%. Which of the following nursing interventions is indicated?

A. Extend the patient's neck and notify the healthcare provider immediately

B. Lay the patient supine and call the healthcare provider immediately

C. Hyper-oxygenate for one minute and then suction the patient's endotracheal tube. Call the healthcare provider if equal breath sounds are not heard after suctioning.

D. Reposition the endotracheal tube 1-2 inches deeper and call the healthcare provider

Rationale:

Correct answer: A

Unequal breath sounds after oral endotracheal intubation suggests the tube is in the right mainstem bronchus. If placed properly, the tube should be centrally located, 5 cm above the carina. The healthcare provider should be notified to reposition the tube.

Flexing and extending the patient's neck can facilitate 2 cm of movement in either direction. (Flexion causes the tube to move downward; extension facilitates movement of the tube upward). The nurse should extend the neck to help the tube move upward slightly, call the healthcare provider, and continue to monitor the patient's oxygenation until the healthcare provider arrives to reposition the tube.

B is incorrect because the patient should not be laid supine. It will be easier to breathe if the head of bed (HOB) is elevated, and the supine position can increase intracranial pressure (ICP) in a decompensating head trauma patient.

C is incorrect because unequal breath sounds are not indicative of secretion accumulation and suctioning will not correct the situation.

D is incorrect because the endotracheal tube does not need to be repositioned deeper, the healthcare provider needs to withdraw the tube and reposition it. It is not within the nurse's scope of practice to extubate, intubate, or reposition an endotracheal tube. An X-ray will need to be performed after repositioning the tube to confirm the position.

42. A patient on the cardiac unit has just had a chest tube placed. The patient refuses to take pain medication and tells the nurse they fear the pain medication will prevent them from being active and taking deep breaths and coughing. What is the best response by the nurse?

A. "The pain medication will make you sleepy."

B. "Pain medication will help control your pain and make it easier to be active and cough."

C. "It's your choice, you don't have to take the pain medication."

D. "I still need you to take the pain medication."

Rationale:

Correct answer: B

"Pain medication will help control your pain and make it easier to be active and cough."

Chest tube insertion is a painful procedure in which a tube is inserted into the pleural space to relieve fluid or air collection. By taking pain medication, the pain will be lessened, making it possible for the patient to be active, breathe deeply and cough effectively. This is necessary to prevent atelectasis and pneumonia.

A is incorrect because there is no guarantee that pain medication will make the patient sleepy, and this statement does not address the patient's concerns.

C is incorrect because, although the patient does have a right to refuse the medication, it is more important for the nurse to provide information about how the pain medication will actually help the patient's breathing. This is patient-focused and will lead to the best possible outcome.

D is incorrect because this statement does not address the patient's fears. The patient ultimately does have a right to refuse the medication and the nurse should not coerce the patient.

43. A patient has a mediastinal chest tube placed during heart surgery and the nurse notes serosanguineous drainage. What are priorities related to the management of this patient's chest tube system in the first 12 hours after surgery?

    A. Monitoring drainage and maintaining tube patency
    B. Monitoring drainage and promoting activity
    C. Maintaining tube patency and promoting airway clearance
    D. Promoting airway clearance and activity

Rationale:

Correct answer: A

Chest tubes are placed during heart surgery to drain blood and fluid that can collect around the heart as a result of the surgery. The chest tube must be monitored for drainage to ensure there is not excessive bleeding necessitating a return to surgery. The chest tube patency must also be maintained to prevent blood and fluid buildup in the pericardial space which would prevent the heart from being able to pump effectively, or cardiac tamponade.

B is incorrect because promoting activity is not an important priority 12 hours after cardiac surgery with chest tube insertion.

C is incorrect because airway clearance is not related to chest tube management.

D is incorrect because activity and airway clearance are not related to chest tube management.

44. A patient with a chest tube for pneumothorax calls the nurse to report the chest tube became dislodged. Which action should the nurse perform immediately?

    A. Call for assistance and check vital signs
    B. Secure the occlusive dressing taped on three sides and notify the healthcare provider
    C. Check vital signs and notify the healthcare provider
    D. Notify the healthcare provider and prepare for insertion of a new chest tube

Rationale:

Correct answer: B

Securing the occlusive dressing over the now open site will prevent air from collecting in the pleural space, which could cause a tension pneumothorax or introduce bacteria. The dressing should be taped on three sides to allow for escape of air as the patient breathes.

A is incorrect because an occlusive dressing should already be at the bedside of any patient with a chest tube in place. The nurse should not need to call for assistance or help in obtaining the dressing. The priority is to apply the dressing taped down on three sides and call the healthcare provider.

C is incorrect because securing the occlusive dressing on three sides is the priority, then calling the healthcare provider.

D is incorrect because although the healthcare provider should be notified and preparation for a new chest tube performed the occlusive dressing needs to be secured first.

45. The healthcare provider is removing a chest tube from a patient with assistance from the nurse. Which of the following statements regarding chest tube removal is incorrect?

    A. The patient must be placed in the prone position for the procedure
    B. Pain medication should be administered 30 minutes prior to the procedure
    C. Emotional support during the procedure is provided by the nurse
    D. The nurse has made suction available

Rationale:

Correct answer: A

Chest tubes are removed after the lung has re-expanded and drainage is minimal. The patient should be supine or in semi-Fowler's for the procedure, not prone.

B is incorrect because it is an appropriate nursing intervention to pre-medicate for pain 30 minutes before removal of a chest tube.

C is incorrect because it is therapeutic for the nurse to provide emotional support during the procedure.

D is incorrect because suction should be available during the removal of a chest tube. The patient should be instructed to *bear down* (Valsalva maneuver) while the healthcare provider removes the clamped chest tube, and then the nurse applies the occlusive dressing.

46. The nurse is caring for a patient with a chest tube that has steady bloody drainage, and the nurse notices clots forming in the drainage tube. What does the nurse do to facilitate drainage of the chest tube?

    A. Strip the chest tube by holding it steady with one hand and pulling gently down the tube with the other
    B. Twist the tube to break up the clots
    C. Tilt the tube back and forth to move the clots down the tube
    D. Notify the healthcare provider to replace the chest tube

Rationale:

Correct answer: C

The chest tube must have patency maintained to prevent ineffective drainage. When clots form in the tube, the tube should be tilted back and forth to keep the clots moving and to facilitate draining into the collection chamber. Allowing the fluid to remain static in the tube can encourage blood clot formation.

A is incorrect because stripping or milking of the tube increases intrathoracic pressure which can cause damage to lung tissue.

B is incorrect because twisting the tube increases intrathoracic pressure, which can cause damage to lung tissue.

D is incorrect because the healthcare provider does not need to be notified unless clots cannot be cleared from the tubing.

47. The nurse on the cardiac unit is caring for a patient after a cardiac catheterization. The nurse finds one of the patient's visitors unresponsive in the bathroom. What is the first action the nurse should perform?

    A. Start chest compressions

    B. Determine DNR status

    C. Call for help

    D. Obtain an automated external defibrillator (AED)

Rationale:

Correct answer: C

If a patient is unresponsive (unarousable, not responding to voice or touch), the next action should be to call for help. This will mobilize people to assist with identification of the individual, resuscitative efforts, and bringing necessary equipment, such as an AED. The nurse should stay with the visitor.

A is incorrect because chest compressions should not be started until lack of a pulse has been confirmed.

B is incorrect because it is unlikely that the nurse has access to a visitor's DNR status documentation. It is more important to call for help. Emergency medical care will be provided to any visitor until DNR information is made available.

D is incorrect because the AED should be brought by another staff member when the nurse calls for help. The nurse should not leave the unresponsive visitor alone.

48. The code team is involved in resuscitating a patient. The AED delivered a shock. What is the next step after a shock has been delivered?

    A. Continue rescue breaths until the AED is ready to deliver another shock

    B. Start an IV and administer normal saline

    C. Check patient's head position for delivery of breaths

    D. Continue CPR for two minutes

Rationale:

Correct answer: D

Chest compressions are imperative to maintain during resuscitative efforts to maintain perfusion of body organs. Interruptions are kept to a minimum and less than 10 seconds each time. After the AED delivers a shock, chest compressions should be immediately resumed and continued for two minutes, with two breaths after every 30 compressions.

A is incorrect because chest compressions should be performed for two minutes before attempting another shock. Rescue breaths, alone, do not provide circulation of blood to the brain.

B is incorrect because chest compressions are more important than starting an IV. If the heart is not beating and the chest is not being manually compressed, infusing normal saline will not circulate through the body and help oxygen reach cells.

C is incorrect because repositioning the head for breaths is important, but chest compressions must be immediately resumed after the AED delivers a shock. After 30 chest compressions are administered, two breaths are delivered. This cycle continues for two minutes or until the AED notifies it is ready to deliver another shock.

49. The nurse is assessing a patient's IV which was placed two days prior. The site is tender when palpated and the surrounding skin is red. Which of the following interventions would be appropriate for the nurse to perform?

   A. Change the IV site dressing
   B. Discontinue the IV and insert a new IV proximal to the original site
   C. Flush the IV to check for patency and administer scheduled antibiotics
   D. Notify the healthcare provider

Rationale:

Correct answer: B

Redness and tenderness at an IV site are symptoms of phlebitis or inflammation of the vein. The IV must be discontinued and a new IV started at another site. This prevents further harm and also allows for IV access for infusion of necessary medications. Other symptoms of phlebitis include heat, swelling, and redness that travels up the path of the vein. Moist, warm compresses are used to treat phlebitis.

A is incorrect because simply changing the IV site dressing will not resolve phlebitis.

C is incorrect because flushing the IV to assess patency and administering ordered antibiotics may worsen phlebitis. Some antibiotics can be extremely caustic if infused into an IV that has already caused tissue damage. The integrity of the IV site must be confirmed before any medications are infused through the IV.

D is incorrect because notifying the healthcare provider about phlebitis is a good action, but the nurse should focus on the patient first. The old IV should be removed and a new IV started before calling the healthcare provider.

50. A patient has just had a peripherally inserted central catheter (PICC) placed and an X-ray performed to confirm placement. The nurse knows the radiologist report should state the tip of the PICC should be located where?

    A. Inferior vena cava
    B. Basilic vein
    C. Cephalic vein
    D. Superior vena cava

Rationale:

Correct answer: D

A peripherally inserted central catheter (PICC) is placed in the upper arm via the basilic or cephalic vein, and when placed correctly, the tip should lie in the superior vena cava just above the right atrium of the heart. PICC lines are used for long-term IV therapy.

A is incorrect because a PICC line would not reach the inferior vena cava, which returns venous blood to the right atrium of the heart.

B is incorrect because the basilic vein is where a PICC is inserted. The basilic vein travels up the forearm to the axilla.

C is incorrect because the cephalic vein is where a PICC is inserted. The cephalic vein runs up the lateral side of the arm from the hand to the shoulder.

51. A patient with a history of right mastectomy needs an IV placed for IV fluid therapy. The patient's veins are more palpable on her right hand, and the patient is left-handed. Where does the nurse place the IV?

    A. Right hand
    B. Left lower arm
    C. Where the patient prefers
    D. Right antecubital

Rationale:

Correct answer: B

When a mastectomy is performed, oftentimes the axillary lymph nodes on the affected side are also removed. This means the patient has less drainage pathways for fluid to move out of the arm. Finger sticks, blood pressure measurements, and IVs should be avoided on the affected side for the rest of the patient's life. Since this patient has had a mastectomy on the right, placing the IV on the right side is contraindicated as it could cause lymphedema. Because of this, the IV should be placed in the left lower arm, even though it is the patient's dominant hand.

A is incorrect because the right side is contraindicated for prevention of lymphedema.

C is incorrect because although patient preference is sometimes considered for IV placement, the post-mastectomy patient must not have an IV placed on the affected side.

D is incorrect because the right side is contraindicated for prevention of lymphedema.

52. A patient has a unit of packed red blood cells infusing when they begin complaining of itching and exhibiting facial flushing. The nurse stops the infusion and checks vital signs. What additional intervention should the nurse perform?

   A. Hang a new IV setup with D_5W to maintain patency of the IV for medication administration
   B. Finish infusing the transfusion left in the tubing and flush with the saline on the Y-site tubing
   C. Begin an infusion of ½ strength normal saline running through the existing blood tubing to keep it patent for diphenhydramine administration
   D. Infuse normal saline with new IV tubing to maintain patency of the IV

Rationale:

Correct answer: D

When a patient experiences a transfusion reaction, it is imperative to maintain IV access, but blood administration tubing must be discontinued so the patient does not receive any more of the donor blood that caused the reaction. The blood bag and tubing should be kept and sent to the blood bank for analysis of what could have caused the reaction. Supportive care includes oxygen, normal saline, diphenhydramine, and potentially corticosteroids. The doctor should be notified immediately.

A is incorrect because D_5W is not used to maintain patency of an IV after a blood transfusion reaction.

B is incorrect because the transfusion has been stopped. It is important that the nurse does not allow any more of the blood to infuse into the patient as this can worsen the reaction.

C is incorrect because the IV tubing must be changed when a blood reaction is suspected, and ½ strength normal saline is not an appropriate fluid to hang after stopping a blood transfusion.

53. The nurse is caring for four patients on the understaffed medical-surgical unit. The nurse is falling behind on the daily schedule. Which of the following tasks cannot be delegated to the UAP?

   A. Nutritional screening
   B. Blood glucose measurement for a newly diagnosed type 2 diabetes patient

C. Feeding a patient with chronic kidney disease

D. Pulse oximetry measurement

Rationale:

Correct answer: A

Unlicensed assistive personnel (UAP) cannot perform assessments or screenings. These are tasks that require the skill of an RN. The nutritional screening, which involves a combination of objective and subjective data, is the responsibility of the nurse. This information helps the nurse determine an individual's nutrition and growth patterns.

B is incorrect because the UAP can perform blood glucose measurements. A newly diagnosed type 2 diabetes patient will require the RN to perform the patient education regarding the glucose level and treatment needed, but the glucometer measurement itself can be delegated.

C is incorrect because the UAP can feed stable patients who are not at risk for aspiration. If the patient has dysphagia or difficulty chewing, the RN is responsible for assessment during mealtime. A patient with chronic kidney disease is not likely to have difficulty chewing or swallowing, so this is a task that can be delegated.

D is incorrect because the UAP can perform pulse oximetry measurements. Any finding less than 95% should be reported to the RN immediately. If the pulse oximetry reading is normal, the UAP can document it in the patient's chart.

54. A patient on the medical unit is on aspiration precautions and is being fed by the nurse. Which of the following is not a priority to prevent aspiration during mealtimes?

    A. Monitor pulse oximetry during feeding
    B. Sit the patient up at 45 degrees for feeding
    C. Maintain suction set-up at the bedside
    D. Delegate the UAP to perform oral care before and after meals

Rationale:

Correct answer: B

Aspiration occurs when a patient has difficulty swallowing, which allows food and fluids to enter the trachea. The head of bed should be elevated to 90 degrees during feeding and kept at 45 degrees at all other times. Risk factors for aspiration include history of dysphagia and aspiration, altered mental status, drug and alcohol overdose, anesthesia, supine position, neurologic conditions, and diseases that cause generalized weakness and prolonged intubation.

A is incorrect because pulse oximetry is necessary during mealtimes. If the patient is aspirating during the meal, the nurse would expect to see the oxygen saturation level decrease.

C is incorrect because this is an appropriate action. Suction equipment should be available at the bedside within the nurse's reach during feeding and throughout the aspiration precautions.

D is incorrect because this is an appropriate measure to take to prevent aspiration. The UAP can perform oral care. Before meals, oral care will clean the mouth and remove any excess oral secretions to allow for optimal chewing and swallowing of the meal. After feedings, oral care will remove any excess food that the patient may still have in the oral cavity, reducing the likelihood of aspiration complications after the meal has been completed.

55. The nurse in the clinic is performing nutritional assessments on four clients. Which of the following statements by a client requires immediate follow-up by the nurse?

    A. "I've lost 10 pounds in the past month."
    B. "I eat more fruits and vegetables now."
    C. "I try to exercise, but it's difficult to find the time."
    D. "I usually eat three or four meals a day."

Rationale:

Correct answer: A

Adult weight is generally stable, and a 10-pound weight loss in one month is a critical indicator the nurse needs to follow up with this patient. For patients trying to decrease their body weight, the Centers for Disease Control and Prevention suggests a safe weight loss at a rate of 1-2 pounds per week. Losing weight at a pace of 3 or more pounds per week can cause lethargy, dizziness, diarrhea, constipation, and dehydration. This is especially true in older adults.

B is incorrect because increasing fruit and vegetable intake is beneficial for providing adequate intake of fiber and other essential nutrients. This can also be helpful for managing cardiovascular disease and decreasing risk factors for many other diseases and complications.

C is incorrect because excessive weight loss is a greater concern. Regular exercise is important as well, and the nurse should follow up with this patient second, but exercise isn't as closely related to the nutritional assessment as weight loss.

D is incorrect because eating 3-4 meals a day is healthy.

56. A patient is admitted to the medical-surgical floor, and the nurse finds a decreased gag reflex during assessment. The healthcare provider has ordered a full liquid diet for the patient. Which of the following actions by the nurse is most important?

    A. Put the patient on NPO status and call the healthcare provider
    B. Allow the patient to eat a meal on the ordered diet and observe for complications
    C. Make sure the head of bed is elevated at mealtime
    D. Put the patient on a clear liquid diet

Rationale:

Correct answer: A

If a patient has a decreased gag reflex, this puts the patient at risk for aspiration. The patient should be NPO until a swallow evaluation can be performed.

B is incorrect because the patient is at risk for aspiration. Decreased gag reflex should be reported to the healthcare provider and the nurse should anticipate a change in the diet ordered. A full liquid diet should not be provided to a patient with a decreased gag reflex.

C is incorrect because the patient is at risk whether or not the head of the bed is elevated.

D is incorrect because the patient is at risk for aspiration. Liquids should not be given PO to this patient. The safest option is to keep the patient NPO until the healthcare provider is notified of the decreased gag reflex and orders a new diet.

57. A patient is experiencing dysphagia after a stroke. Which of the following foods is inappropriate for the nurse to offer the patient?

    A. Minced meat
    B. Custard
    C. Whole milk
    D. Steamed winter squash

Rationale:

Correct answer: C

Any type of milk is a thin liquid that should be avoided as a beverage in a patient with dysphagia. Patients experiencing dysphagia are at risk for aspiration and have an easier time swallowing soft textures. The patient with dysphagia post-stroke should be on a soft diet. Thin liquids and foods that require a lot of chewing put the patient at risk for aspirating their meal. Milk can be added to thicker items, such as soups and smoothies.

A is incorrect because on a soft diet, all meat and fish should be shredded or minced and served with sufficient gravy to aid in swallowing.

B is incorrect because custard is an appropriate dessert for a patient with dysphagia. Custard can be made with fresh eggs and milk to provide additional calcium and protein. This boosts nutrient intake and adds variety to the diet without compromising swallowing.

D is incorrect because squash is a versatile vegetable offering many nutrients such as vitamin A, vitamin C, iron, and carbohydrates. When steamed, this vegetable is very easy to mash, making it acceptable for a soft diet.

58. The nurse is caring for a patient with a ruptured cerebral aneurysm. The patient is DNR status. After inserting a nasogastric tube into the patient for enteral feedings, which of the following placement verification methods is most appropriate before the nurse begins using the tube?

    A. Observing the color and amount of fluid withdrawn from the nasogastric tube
    B. pH testing of fluid withdrawn from the tube
    C. Auscultating an air bolus over the left upper abdominal quadrant
    D. X-ray of the chest and abdomen

Rationale:

Correct answer: D

When placing a nasogastric or orogastric tube for enteral feedings, an X-ray of the tube must be performed before instilling anything into the tube. The tube must be confirmed for placement by a healthcare provider before it can be used to instill medications, provide fluid, or administer feeding.

A is incorrect because observing the color of fluid withdrawn from the tube is not sufficient for tube placement verification. The color of the fluid is generally green or brown but can vary, depending on what was ingested recently. The amount of fluid is the *residual* which confirms gastric emptying but does not guarantee placement.

B is incorrect because after initial placement of a gastric feeding tube, an X-ray is the standard for verifying placement. pH testing is used to confirm placement of an established feeding tube but is not appropriate for confirmation after initial placement. The pH of the stomach should be low: 1-4, from hydrochloric acid secreted by the gastric mucosa. The pH of the duodenum will be higher, due to bicarbonate from pancreatic juice secreted into the duodenum.

C is incorrect because auscultation over the left upper quadrant for an air bolus is no longer the standard of care for feeding tube placement. Research has shown that if the tube is accidentally inserted into the left lung, an air bolus pushed through the tube may still be heard over the left upper quadrant. If this method is used to check placement, the risk is that the nurse will inadvertently insert medications or instill tube feedings into the lung.

59. The nurse is caring for a patient diagnosed with lymphocytic leukemia. The patient is receiving enteral feedings via nasogastric tube. The patient complains of abdominal cramping and has had two episodes of diarrhea, measuring 200 mL and 250 mL each. Before notifying the healthcare provider, which information does the nurse need to collect?

    A. Patency of the nasogastric tube
    B. If the enteral feedings contain sorbitol
    C. If the patient has a latex allergy
    D. Oxygen saturation

Rationale:

Correct answer: B

Enteral feedings can contain sorbitol, an artificial sweetener that can cause diarrhea. If the cause of the diarrhea is the sorbitol, the enteral feeding needs to be changed, by order from the healthcare provider to a formula that does not contain sorbitol.

A is incorrect because patency of the nasogastric tube will not contribute to diarrhea. Diarrhea will not be a result of an occluded tube (which would decrease the amount of food or fluid that reaches the intestines).

C is incorrect because a latex allergy is unlikely and will not cause diarrhea. NG tubes often are not made of latex. They are usually made from polyurethane or silicone.

D is incorrect because although oxygen saturation should be monitored with every vital sign assessment, this is a piece of data that is unrelated to the diarrhea.

60. A 75-year-old patient with a history of constipation is receiving enteral feedings via nasogastric tube. Upon assessing the patient, the nurse observes diminished bowel sounds. Which action should the nurse perform first?

    A. Assess the patient for nausea, abdominal pain, and abdominal distention
    B. Call the healthcare provider to request a stool softener
    C. Obtain the patient's weight
    D. Stop the enteral feeding

Rationale:

Correct answer: A

Given the patient's history and diminished bowel sounds, it is important to assess for nausea, abdominal pain, and abdominal distention and compare them to the patient's baseline and recent history. This is valuable information that can ascertain whether the patient is constipated and needs a stool softener. Complications of enteral feedings include cramping, vomiting, and diarrhea more commonly than constipation.

B is incorrect because the nurse needs to perform an abdominal assessment before notifying the healthcare provider or using a pharmacologic intervention such as a stool softener. Unnecessary stool softeners can cause diarrhea, dehydration, and dependence.

C is incorrect because weight is an indicator of fluid status, not bowel patterns.

D is incorrect because diminished bowel sounds are not a contraindication to enteral feedings.

61. The nurse is caring for patients on the renal unit receiving enteral feedings. The nurse identifies which of the following is inappropriate for patients receiving enteral feedings?

    A. Use clean technique to insert nasogastric tubes
    B. Keep enteral feeding solutions at room temperature
    C. Handle the feeding system using aseptic technique
    D. Change the tubing with every feeding

Rationale:

Correct answer: D

Enteral feeding is used to deliver nutrients into the gastrointestinal system (stomach or intestine) to a patient who is otherwise unable to take PO food and fluids. Tubing should be changed every 24 hours to prevent bacterial growth but does not need to be changed with each feeding.

A is incorrect because this is appropriate nursing practice. Clean technique is used to insert a nasogastric tube. The tip of the tube is lubricated with clean water-soluble jelly. Clean tap water is offered to drink as the tube is passed through the nose into the stomach.

B is incorrect because keeping the enteral feeding at room temperature reduces discomfort. It is not necessary to chill enteral feedings to prevent bacterial growth. The bag should not be left hanging for more than four hours.

C is incorrect because aseptic technique should be used to prevent infection.

62. The nurse on the medical-surgical unit is caring for patients receiving parenteral nutrition. The nurse knows that which of the following is a risk associated with parenteral nutrition?

    A. Bowel obstruction
    B. Pneumonia
    C. Increased albumin levels
    D. Catheter-related bloodstream infections

Rationale:

Correct answer: D

The most common risk associated with short-term parenteral nutrition is catheter-related bloodstream infections. The nurse must take care to use aseptic technique when attaching the tubing to the catheter and sterile technique when changing the central line dressing. Other complications of parenteral nutrition include hyperglycemia, hypoglycemia, fluid volume overload, and air embolism.

A is incorrect because parenteral nutrition is given intravenously and would not contribute to a bowel obstruction. Bowel obstruction is an indication of parenteral nutrition. Bowel obstruction is a contraindication to enteral feedings delivered by feeding tube.

B is incorrect because there is no relation between parenteral nutrition and pneumonia.

C is incorrect because albumin levels are more likely to be decreased.

63. The nurse is caring for patients receiving long-term parenteral nutrition. The nurse knows these patients are at risk for which of the following?

    A. Dehydration
    B. Hypercholesterolemia
    C. Hepatic disease
    D. Renal disease

Rationale:

Correct answer: C

Hepatic disease is associated with bloodstream infections, severe gastrointestinal dysfunction, and long-term parenteral nutrition. Other complications related to long-term parenteral nutrition include metabolic bone disease and increased triglycerides.

A is incorrect because fluid volume overload is a risk of parenteral nutrition, not dehydration.

B is incorrect because the lipids in parenteral nutrition do not contain cholesterol.

D is incorrect because there is no connection between long-term parenteral nutrition and renal function.

64. The nurse receives an order from the healthcare provider for an external condom catheter. Which of the following interventions by the nurse will prevent skin irritation and infection?

    A. Apply the condom sheath so the end of the catheter is 3-to-5 inches from the tip of the penis

    B. Shave the pubic area to prevent adherence to the condom or pulling during removal of the catheter

    C. Clean the area before applying the condom catheter

    D. Apply the condom sheath tightly with tape to secure it in place

Rationale:

Correct answer: C

Providing hygiene to the area before applying the condom catheter will prevent skin irritation and infection. Mild soap and water are used, and the nurse should take care to dry the area thoroughly before applying the condom catheter. Water-soluble lubricant may be needed to facilitate the procedure.

A is incorrect because there should be 1-to-2 inches between the tip of the penis and the catheter. If too much space is left between the tip of the penis and the condom catheter, this could lead to urine leakage, which can contribute to skin breakdown.

B is incorrect because shaving may increase skin irritation. Excess hair near the base of the penis should be clipped so it does not get caught in the condom or attachment.

D is incorrect because the condom should be secure but not tight, as this can reduce blood flow to the penis.

65. A patient with an indwelling urinary catheter calls the nurse complaining of pain in the lower abdomen. When the nurse assesses the patient, lower abdominal tenderness and distention are noted. The patient has had no urine output over the last hour. What is the first action the nurse should perform?

    A. Irrigate the catheter with saline or sterile water

    B. Assess the drainage tubing for kinks

    C. Encourage the patient to drink water

    D. Discontinue the urinary catheter

Rationale:

Correct answer: B

The first intervention the nurse should perform is to assess the urinary catheter drainage tube for any kinks. There may be some type of obstruction in the catheter, and problems with drainage are most commonly attributed to kinks in the tubing.

A is incorrect because irrigation may be indicated in the case of obstruction, but the tubing should be checked for kinks first. The nurse should use the least invasive measures first, such as assessing the tubing for proper outflow.

C is incorrect because PO intake should not be encouraged if a catheter obstruction is suspected. PO fluids will increase urine formation, which can be detrimental and can increase pain as the fluid moves from the ureters to the urethra.

D is incorrect because the source of the obstruction should be identified first. If the obstruction can be relieved, the patient may not need the catheter to be removed. The nurse should attempt the least-invasive measures first. Discontinuing the catheter will not allow for appropriate drainage of urine and inserting a new catheter risks infection.

66. The nurse is caring for patients on the medical-surgical unit. Which of the following patients is a candidate for a urinary catheter?

    A. Patient with a stage I pressure ulcer who is incontinent
    B. Patient who is incontinent if unassisted to the bedside commode
    C. Patient with high post-void residuals
    D. Patient who is incontinent of urine

Rationale:

Correct answer: C

Urinary catheters are not appropriate for every patient as their use can contribute to catheter associated urinary tract infections (CAUTI). Evidence-based guidelines support the use of urinary catheters in patients who experience retention.

A is incorrect because guidelines do not support the use of an indwelling catheter with a stage I pressure ulcer. If the pressure ulcer is open (stage II-IV), urinary catheterization is indicated.

B is incorrect because requiring assistance with toileting is not an indication for a catheter. The nurse should assure that adequate assistance is available to help the patient to the bedside commode when required.

D is incorrect because urinary incontinence is not an indication for a catheter.

67. The nurse is caring for a patient experiencing hematuria who had a three-way urinary catheter with continuous bladder irrigation (CBI) placed. The patient calls the nurse to complain of lower abdominal pain. What is the first intervention the nurse should perform?

   A. Increase the flow rate of the CBI
   B. Check the drainage tubing for kinks
   C. Decrease the flow rate of the CBI
   D. Check the patient's temperature

Rationale:

Correct answer: B

Continuous bladder irrigation (CBI) is utilized in patients who experience obstruction due to cancer, bleeding, or infection. This patient most likely has an obstruction to drainage, which would cause lower abdominal pain due to bladder distention. There should consistently be more fluid in the drainage bag than the flow rate of the CBI. The nurse should check the tubing for kinks to ensure proper drainage. Relieving a kink will provide the most immediate pain relief.

A is incorrect because increasing the flow rate will contribute to additional pain and distention.

C is incorrect because decreasing the flow rate may decrease the pain but will not treat the problem.

D is incorrect because checking the patient's temperature will have no effect on drainage or pain.

68. A patient is admitted to the emergency room for stool impaction. The nurse knows that digital removal increases risk for unintended vagus nerve stimulation and therefore, should monitor the patient for which of the following?

   A. Urinary incontinence
   B. Increased heart rate
   C. Abdominal cramping
   D. Decreased heart rate

Rationale:

Correct answer: D

Digital removal is commonly performed for stool impaction. Because the vagus nerve is close to the rectum, the risk for stimulating it is high, which may lead to a drop in heart rate.

A is incorrect because stimulation of the vagus nerve does not cause urinary incontinence.

B is incorrect because stimulation of the vagus nerve causes bradycardia, not an increased heart rate.

C is incorrect because stimulation of the vagus nerve does not cause abdominal cramping.

Note: This is different from intentional medical vagus nerve stimulation used to treat epilepsy.

69. The nurse is inserting a nasogastric tube in a patient experiencing nausea and vomiting due to bowel obstruction. The nurse knows that the patient is asked to swallow during the procedure because this causes:

   A. Stimulation of the gag reflex
   B. Closing of the upper airway to direct the nasogastric tube to the stomach
   C. Easier passing of the nasogastric tube through the nasal passage
   D. Distraction of the patient during insertion of the nasogastric tube

Rationale:

Correct answer: B

Swallowing during insertion of a nasogastric tube closes off the upper airway to help direct the tube to the stomach and away from the lungs.

A is incorrect because insertion of a nasogastric tube causes stimulation of the gag reflex and swallowing does not prevent this.

C is incorrect because swallowing does not affect passage of the nasogastric tube through the nasal passage. Swallowing facilitates passage of the tube through the pharynx and into the esophagus.

D is incorrect because swallowing does not distract the patient from the procedure.

70. The nurse cares for a patient who had small intestine surgery for bowel obstruction. The patient had a nasogastric tube placed in the operating room. The nasogastric tube is attached to suction for gastric decompression. The patient calls the nurse complaining of nausea, and upon assessment, the nurse finds the patient's abdomen is distended. Resistance is met when the nasogastric tube is irrigated. What is the next action the nurse should take?

   A. Irrigate the tube again with normal saline
   B. Turn the patient onto their left side
   C. Advance the nasogastric tube three inches
   D. Switch the wall suction to continuous

Rationale:

Correct answer: B

Gastric decompression is used to keep the stomach empty in a patient with bowel obstruction. It is important to remove gastric juice from the stomach so that it does not empty into the small intestine. Suction pressure and position can cause a nasogastric tube to become stuck to the wall of the stomach. Turning the patient onto their left side can naturally reposition the tube, making it easier to flush and regain suction. Proper suction is needed to maintain gastric decompression.

A is incorrect because irrigating the tube again is not necessary. Resistance has already been identified, so irrigating again will not fix the problem.

C is incorrect because it is not within the nurse's scope of practice to advance a tube that has been surgically placed.

D is incorrect because it is not within the nurse's scope of practice to change the suction method. Continuous suction applied to a nasogastric tube can be irritating to the gastric mucosa and can cause a gastric bleed.

71. The nurse is caring for a patient with a new sigmoid colostomy and is educating them on care of the ostomy at home. The patient demonstrates a need for further instruction when they make which statement?

    A. "I should use warm water to clean the skin around the stoma."
    B. "I will eat my normal, well-balanced diet."
    C. "Every time I change my pouch, I need to look at the skin for irritation."
    D. "I will measure the stoma each time and call the doctor if the shape or size changes."

Rationale:

Correct answer: D

A new stoma is edematous when it is first created, and the swelling will decrease over 4-to-6 weeks. The patient will have to buy different fitting bags as the swelling decreases. A decrease in the size and shape of the stoma is not indicative to report to the healthcare provider.

A is incorrect because warm water and mild soap should be used to wash around the stoma.

B is incorrect because the stool is soft and formed when a balanced diet is consumed. The patient does not need to make dietary modifications as long as they consume a well-balanced diet and adequate fluid.

C is incorrect because the patient should be taught to observe the skin for any irritation each time the pouch is changed.

72. The risk management nurse explains the significance of Do Not Resuscitate (DNR) status in the surgical area during an in-service for the new staff. Which of the following statements regarding DNR orders is true?

    A. DNR applies in the post-operative period only, but the patient may be resuscitated during the surgery if needed.
    B. DNR is automatically suspended during and immediately after surgery
    C. The surgeon should discuss DNR with the patient and family
    D. Patients with DNR are not candidates for surgery

Rationale:

Correct answer: C

Whenever a patient has a DNR, the surgeon should discuss maintaining or modifying DNR for during the surgical procedure and invasive procedures. Once discussed, the plan for the DNR is documented in the patient's medical record. Some patients will suspend the DNR during the surgery but specifically request that resuscitation measures will not be implemented in the recovery period. Unless these specific wishes are documented, DNR stands and the patient should not be resuscitated under any circumstances.

A is incorrect because DNR applies to care of the patient before, during, and after surgery.

B is incorrect because DNR is never automatically suspended.

D is incorrect because DNR does not mean *do not treat*. DNR status does not impact whether a patient is a candidate for surgery.

73. The post-anesthesia care unit (PACU) nurse is caring for a patient following hip replacement surgery and notes drainage on the dressing. Which of the following interventions should the nurse perform?

    A. This is expected; document that drainage is noted
    B. Mark the dressing by tracing the drainage
    C. Remove the dressing and assess how much bleeding is occurring
    D. Notify the surgeon immediately

Rationale:

Correct answer: B

Some amount of bleeding is expected after hip replacement surgery, but the PACU nurse should trace around the drainage noted so that on follow-up assessment, the amount of bleeding and/or drainage can be easily identified.

A is incorrect because the drainage needs to be measured and marked with a pen or marker so that it can be monitored.

C is incorrect because the first post-op dressing should not be removed by the nurse.

D is incorrect because the surgeon does not need to be notified for a small amount of drainage.

Select All That Apply

74. The charge nurse on the medical-surgical unit has made assignments for the nursing team. The charge nurse knows which team members are responsible for coordinating discharge for a patient who has recovered after hip surgery. (Select all that apply):

    A. Primary nurse
    B. Social worker
    C. Unlicensed assistive personnel (UAP)
    D. Healthcare provider
    E. Family members

    Rationale:

    Correct answer: A, B, D

    The discharge plan is very important and requires the input of many healthcare professionals for the best patient outcomes and to prevent readmissions. The primary nurse caring for the patient knows the patient best and is responsible for the discharge teaching. The social worker should also be included as they can help identify resources in the patient's home location. The healthcare provider is a part of the discharge process and is responsible for ordering the medications and treatments as well as follow-up visits.

    C is incorrect because the UAP is focused on completing tasks and does not have input regarding the patient's discharge plan.

    E is incorrect because the family members do not contribute to the discharge plan, although they may be an integral part of following the plan.

75. The nurse is documenting care on the medical unit. When the narrative nursing note is documented, which of the following is important? (Select all that apply):

    A. Document immediately after care is provided
    B. Record any information other staff members provide
    C. Each entry starts with date and time

D. Perform all documentation at the end of the shift

E. Errors on paper documentation have a single line drawn through them

Rationale:

Correct answer: A, C, E

Care and interventions must be documented immediately following provision of that care. There are times when it is appropriate to document during care, such as vital signs, and intake and output. Every entry should have date and time for the most accuracy and future recall. Errors on paper documentation should have a single line drawn through them as well as initials of the person documenting. This allows for the erroneous information to still be legible.

B is incorrect because information provided by others should be documented by those providing the information.

D is incorrect because documentation should be completed throughout the shift, as tasks are performed and assessments are made. This provides for better recall and more accurate documentation in the legal patient record. Waiting until the end of shift to record assessments may lead to inadvertent omission of important patient details. Documentation should occur immediately after care has been provided.

76. The nurse is caring for a confused patient and needs to check the patient's axillary temperature. Which of the following nursing actions would best provide accurate temperature measurement? (Select all that apply):

    A. Dry the axilla before checking the temperature
    B. Hold the temperature probe steady in the axilla
    C. Position the patient supine
    D. Make sure the patient has had nothing by mouth in the last 15 minutes
    E. Communicate with the patient while checking the temperature

Rationale:

Correct answer: A, B, E

Axillary temperature is best for a patient who is confused in order to obtain an accurate temperature. Drying the axilla of any perspiration will ensure better contact with the temperature probe for a more accurate result. Holding the probe in place also ensures better contact with the axilla. Talking with the confused patient can keep them calm and distract them from the probe in their axilla.

C is incorrect because it is unnecessary to place the patient supine for an axillary temperature. A confused patient should be kept with the head of bed elevated and the nurse should provide frequent reorientation.

D is incorrect because nothing to eat or drink for 15 minutes applies to oral temperature, not axillary.

77. A patient is placed on isolation precautions for MRSA pneumonia. The nurse will intervene when the UAP does which of the following? (Select all that apply):

    A.   Minimizes talking with the patient to promote rest
    B.   Uses an N-95 respirator mask when caring for the patient
    C.   Encourages the patient to use the incentive spirometer (IS) 10 times each hour
    D.   Delivers the meal tray to the patient's room
    E.   Provides personal protective equipment (PPE) to visiting family members

Rationale:

Correct answer: A, B

Patients on isolation precautions are at risk for social isolation and depression. All members of the healthcare team should interact with the patient as much as possible when in the patient's room to prevent depression. MRSA requires contact precautions (gown, gloves when in close contact with the patient). An N-95 respirator mask is indicated for a patient on airborne precautions.

C is incorrect because this is an appropriate action. The patient with pneumonia needs to use the IS 10 times hourly while awake to prevent atelectasis. The nurse is responsible for teaching the patient how to use the IS, but the UAP can encourage the use of the equipment.

D is incorrect because it is appropriate for the UAP to deliver a meal into the room of a patient on contact precautions. The patient should not be allowed to leave the room unless needed for specific tests or procedures.

E is incorrect because this is an appropriate action. Any visitors who are going to come into close contact with the patient should wear PPE to protect themselves from the MRSA infection.

78. The nurse is learning about which procedures require sterile technique and which require clean technique. Which of the following procedures require sterile technique? (Select all that apply):

    A.   Urinary catheter insertion
    B.   Nasogastric tube insertion
    C.   Nasotracheal suctioning
    D.   Central line dressing change

E.   Peripheral IV insertion

Rationale:

Correct answer: A, C, D

Insertion of a urinary catheter, nasotracheal suctioning, and central line dressing change all require the use of sterile technique. The lines being inserted enter what is considered a sterile body cavity, and any introduction of microorganisms may lead to infection.

B is incorrect because nasogastric (NG) tube insertion does not require sterile technique. Clean technique is appropriate for NG tube insertion. Microorganisms introduced would likely be destroyed by hydrochloric acid in gastric juice.

E is incorrect because peripheral IV insertion and dressing changes do not require sterile technique, although the IV catheter must be kept sterile before insertion.

79. A patient is having a traction boot applied to the left lower extremity by the nurse for Buck's traction. Which of the following actions should the nurse perform during the procedure? (Select all that apply):
    A.   Shave the lower left leg
    B.   Ensure a snug fit of the boot
    C.   Place a pad in the heel of the boot
    D.   Slowly and gently apply the weight at the foot of the bed
    E.   Reassess neurovascular status of the affected foot distal to the traction

Rationale:

Correct answer: B, D, E

Buck's traction is applied to a fractured extremity in order to realign the bones. The boot is applied snugly to the affected leg, and a weight is attached to a rope attached to the heel of the boot.

Neurovascular status of the affected foot is assessed distal to traction once the weight is applied and at regular intervals according to facility policy.

A is incorrect because shaving may cause microvascular trauma which can become inflamed and cause irritation and even infection.

C is incorrect because when the boot is applied properly, the heel sits elevated, so padding is not added to prevent pressure on the heel.

80. A patient calls the nurse after application of an arm cast complaining of pain and swelling. Which of the following interventions should the nurse take? (Select all that apply):

A. Assess cast tightness

B. Elevate the arm on a pillow

C. Perform neurovascular checks every 15 minutes

D. Lower the arm with the cast

E. Notify the healthcare provider and administer analgesics

F. Apply bags of ice to the cast

Rationale:

Correct answer: A, B, C, F

Pain and swelling after cast application indicates swelling under the cast. The arm should be elevated to decrease edema and promote venous return. The nurse should check neurovascular status often to determine if circulation is impaired. Cast tightness will indicate how much swelling and edema are present.

D is incorrect because the arm should be elevated.

E is incorrect because the healthcare provider should be notified, but analgesics will not relieve the edema and could mask the worsening of symptoms. Analgesics should be withheld until compartment syndrome has been ruled out and a decision has been made about whether the cast needs to be removed.

81. The nurse manager is documenting Quality and Safety Education for Nurses (QSEN) skills for competency for the nurses on the unit. Which of the following behaviors demonstrates competency of QSEN? (Select all that apply):

    A. The nurses use memory recall to remember which of three patients is due for analgesic administration in 30 minutes

    B. A patient is placed on a bed alarm system by a nurse who has not received training on the system

    C. A nurse assesses a patient's fall risk using evidence-based guidelines

    D. The nurse includes the occurrence of a patient fall during shift report

    E. Inservice opportunities offer nurses opportunities to practice new skills in a simulation lab

Rationale:

Correct answer: C, D, E

Quality and Safety Education for Nurses (QSEN) was designed to develop quality and safety competencies for nursing focused on patient-centered care, evidence-based practice, safety, teamwork and collaboration, quality improvement, and informatics. Evidence-based guidelines should be used to determine risk for falls, and all patient safety issues should be communicating to the next shift to ensure safe care is provided. Simulated experiences have been shown to increase nurse competency in practicing new skills.

A is incorrect because memory recall is not a QSEN category.

B is incorrect because use of new equipment without proper training does not meet QSEN.

82. The nurse has applied bilateral upper extremity restraints to prevent a belligerent patient from injuring themselves and the staff. In order to minimize vulnerability and protect the patient, which of the following approaches to restraint application are patient-centered? (Select all that apply):

    A. Evaluate the meaning of restraints according to the patient's family
    B. Obtain consent from the patient before applying restraints
    C. Collaborate with the patient's family in order to accommodate cultural beliefs regarding restraints
    D. Identify whether the patient prefers a soft wrist restraint or a mitten restraint
    E. Assess circulation and offer a snack, beverage, and toileting opportunity every three hours

Rationale:

Correct answer: A, C, D

Patient-centered care involves consideration of cultural perspectives and meanings of interventions in healthcare. A restraint may be perceived as punishment. Restraint type preference should be considered as well. Even a belligerent patient may be able to indicate preference of which type of restraint is used. This helps the patient to maintain some sense of control over their situation. When possible, the nurse should include views and opinions of patient and family for patient-centered care.

B is incorrect because the nurse cannot obtain consent from a belligerent patient.

E is incorrect because food, drink, and use of the commode should be offered every two hours. Circulation should be checked every 30 minutes.

83. The nurse on the medical-surgical unit is assessing patients for wound healing. Which of the following patients are at risk for delayed wound healing? (Select all that apply):

    A. Patient with an elevated white cell count and a surgical wound that has yellow drainage
    B. Cancer patient receiving cortisol
    C. Older adult with prescribed increased vitamin C intake
    D. Trauma patient with a clean, open wound treated with a moist dressing
    E. Patient with an upper respiratory infection taking echinacea

Rationale:

Correct answer: A, B

The surgical wound with yellow drainage is most likely infected, as evidenced by the elevated white cell count, which would delay wound healing. The cancer patient is taking cortisol, a glucocorticoid hormone. This medication is an anti-inflammatory, which may delay wound healing and can mask signs of infection.

C is incorrect because vitamin C will promote wound healing.

D is incorrect because moist dressings can promote wound healing.

E is incorrect because echinacea can promote wound healing.

84. The nurse is caring for a patient on the medical-surgical unit who is hearing impaired. Which of the following techniques would be most appropriate by the nurse to facilitate communication? (Select all that apply):

   A. Increase the volume at which the nurse speaks
   B. Decrease the speed at which the nurse speaks
   C. Always speak to the patient where the patient can see the nurse's face
   D. Use hand gestures to assist in explaining speech
   E. Determine patient's ability to read

Rationale:

Correct answer: B, C, D, E

When caring for a patient that is hearing impaired, the best interventions include speaking slowly in a normal tone and standing where the patient can see the nurse's face. If a patient does not understand, word choice may be changed and hand gestures may be used to enhance understanding, but sometimes the patient needs more time to process the information in order to answer questions.

The nurse may also determine if the patient can read, because communicating in writing may be effective. If the patient has better hearing on one side, the nurse should direct speech toward the side with stronger hearing. The nurse should be sure to keep hands and other objects away from the face when speaking and have the patient repeat statements to ensure the proper information has been heard.

A is incorrect because speaking in a louder tone distorts speech and can make it more difficult to understand. The nurse should speak clearly and slowly but avoid a raised voice.

85. The nurse on the intensive care unit is caring for intubated patients. Which of the following actions by the UAP requires the nurse to intervene? (Select all that apply):

    A. Elevating the head of the bed at 10 degrees

    B. Repositioning the patient every four hours

    C. Providing oral care with chlorhexidine every eight hours

    D. Checking pH to be sure the tip of the feeding tube is in the duodenum

    E. Frequent tracheal suctioning

Rationale:

Correct answer: A, B, D, E

The prevalence of hospital-acquired infection is a significant concern in acutely ill patients. Ventilator-associated pneumonia (VAP) contributes to mortality in patients who are intubated and on the ventilator for more than 24-48 hours. The patient should be repositioned every two hours and the head of bed should be kept elevated at least 30 degrees to prevent VAP and aspiration in intubated patients.

Frequent tracheal suctioning is required to prevent VAP, but the UAP cannot perform tracheal suctioning. If a feeding tube is needed, it is important to keep the end of the tube beyond the pylorus of the stomach to reduce VAP. However, it is not within the UAP's scope of practice to check the placement of the feeding tube.

C is incorrect because this is a good action to prevent VAP. Studies have shown chlorhexidine to be effective and safe for oral care in intubated patients to prevent VAP as it kills oral bacteria. It is within the UAP's scope of practice to provide oral care with chlorhexidine solution.

86. The nurse on the intensive care unit is caring for patients with impaired airways. Which of the following statements are true in safe maintenance of patient airways? (Select all that apply):

    A. Respiratory assessment has two components: respiratory rate and oxygen saturation level

    B. Risk of aspiration is a factor when enteral feeding tubes are present

    C. Airway equipment must be evaluated for functionality before each use

    D. Review of previous shift information is irrelevant for care of the patient on the current shift

    E. After removing soiled tracheostomy ties, the nurse should carefully hold the tracheostomy tube in place while applying the new ties

Rationale:

Correct answer: B, C

Ventilator-associated pneumonia (VAP) is a lung infection that is contracted when a patient is on a ventilator for longer than 24 hours. Implementations to prevent VAP include assessing for risk of aspiration with or without a feeding tube and frequent oral care. It is always important to evaluate airway equipment every shift and before each use when caring for intubated patients.

A is incorrect because respiratory assessment includes respiratory rate, depth of respirations, oxygen saturation, patency of airway, breath sounds, equality of the breath sounds, and respiratory effort.

D is incorrect because reviewing baseline or previous shift documentation is important when caring for a patient.

E is incorrect because old ties should remain in place when the new tracheostomy ties are inserted. This prevents accidental dislodgement of the tracheostomy tube.

87. Cardiopulmonary resuscitation (CPR) is being performed on a patient in the emergency department. Which of the following actions should occur every two minutes during the code procedure? (Select all that apply):

    A. Checking rate of IV fluids
    B. Interrupting chest compressions to switch providers
    C. Analyzing heart rhythm and presence of a pulse
    D. Administration of amiodarone
    E. Provide two breaths

Rationale:

Correct answer: B, C

During a code, the chest compressions should be interrupted every two minutes to switch providers to prevent fatigue and maintain effectiveness of compressions. While chest compressions are stopped, the monitor should be checked for rhythm, and the patient should be assessed for presence of a pulse.

A is incorrect because IV fluids do not need to be checked every two minutes during a code.

D is incorrect because amiodarone is not administered for all codes and is not given every two minutes.

E is incorrect because two breaths are provided for every 30 compressions via bag-valve-mask (BVM) or 8-10 times per minute via endotracheal tube.

88. The purpose of a rapid response team is to (select all that apply):

    A. Provide early intervention to prevent cardiac arrest
    B. Facilitate transfer of a patient to a higher level of care

C. Reduce hospital mortality rate

D. Negate the need for a code blue team

E. Write orders for interventions

Rationale:

Correct answer: A, B, C

The purpose of a rapid response team includes intervening early to prevent cardiac arrest, reduce hospital mortality rates due to early intervention, and to facilitate transfer of a patient to a higher level of care when needed. The RRT fosters collaboration between critical care nurses and medical-surgical nurses in the care of patients through assessment, communication, immediate interventions, support, and education. The RRT may consist of any of the following members of the healthcare team: nurse, physician, intensivist, respiratory therapist, physician assistant, and clinical nurse specialist.

D is incorrect because a rapid response team does not negate the need for a code blue team. If a patient is in cardiac arrest or has no pulse, a code is called. If a patient has a sudden decline in status, the Rapid Response team is called.

E is incorrect because the Rapid Response team cannot write orders and the healthcare provider always needs to be notified of a change in patient status.

89. A patient is placed on a clear liquid diet for gastritis. The nurse knows a clear liquid diet includes (select all that apply):

A. Iced tea

B. Coffee with cream and sweetener

C. Popsicles

D. Beef broth

E. Ice cream

Rationale:

Correct answer: A, C, D

Clear liquids include foods that are liquid at room temperature and are clear in color. They leave little residue and are easily absorbed. Clear liquids are commonly ordered after surgery, before diagnostic procedures, and in patients experiencing diarrhea and vomiting. Coffee and tea (without additives), clear soda, popsicles, Jell-O, water, pulp-free juices, and broth are all considered clear liquids.

B is incorrect because coffee is only allowed on a clear liquid diet if it is served black, without any additives.

E is incorrect because ice cream is not a clear liquid. Ice cream is allowed on a full liquid diet, which also includes cream soups (without particles), milk, milkshakes, and pudding.

90. The nurse is caring for five patients on the medical-surgical floor. All of the patients have been on enteral feeding. Which of these patients have indications for parenteral nutrition? (Select all that apply):

    A. Patient who is scheduled for small intestine surgery
    B. Patient who has chronic high residuals on enteral feedings
    C. Patient who was admitted for acute pancreatitis
    D. Patient who has an intestinal obstruction
    E. Patient who is one day post-operative from lung surgery and is tolerating PO liquids

Rationale:

Correct answer: A, B, C, D

Parenteral nutrition is given intravenously to patients who have significantly altered GI function because it allows for complete nutritional needs to be met while allowing the GI system to rest and recover. Small intestine surgery and bowel obstructions both require time for the gut to rest for several days post-op. Chronic high residuals with enteral feedings indicate that the feedings are not properly moving through the pylorus of the stomach into the small intestine, thus nutrition is not being absorbed. Acute pancreatitis requires NPO status and nothing into the GI tract.

E is incorrect because the patient is tolerating PO liquids, and surgery was not GI in nature. This patient has no indication for a change to parenteral nutrition.

91. A patient has orders from the healthcare provider to discontinue the urinary catheter. Which of the following interventions does the nurse implement? (Select all that apply):

    A. Attach a 5 mL syringe to the balloon inflation port
    B. Allow gravity drainage of the balloon into the syringe
    C. Initiate a bladder diary
    D. Pull the catheter out quickly
    E. Pull back on the syringe plunger with steady force

Rationale:

Correct answer: B, C

Allowing the balloon to drain by gravity into the syringe will prevent ridges from forming on the balloon once deflated. This will prevent damage to the urethra as the urinary catheter is withdrawn.

Once the urinary catheter is withdrawn, the nurse needs to monitor bladder function by documenting a bladder diary. If the patient is unable to void four hours after the urinary catheter is withdrawn, this may indicate a urethral obstruction or urinary retention, and the healthcare provider will need to be notified.

A is incorrect because the size of the syringe used depends on the catheter. The balloon size is indicated on the port and the same size syringe should be used to deflate. Often, the balloon holds 10 mL, so a 5 mL syringe won't fully deflate the balloon.

D is incorrect because the urinary catheter should be withdrawn slowly to prevent damage to the urethra.

E is incorrect because pulling back on the plunger can cause formation of ridges in the catheter balloon.

92. The nurse is caring for a patient with a suprapubic catheter. Which of the following interventions does the nurse provide? (Select all that apply):

    A. Clean the skin around the catheter using sterile technique and a circular motion
    B. Wipe away drainage on the tube down the catheter and close to the insertion site
    C. Assess the insertion site for erythema, edema, tenderness, and discharge
    D. Gently pull on the catheter when cleaning the tube and the insertion site
    E. Deflate the balloon while cleaning the catheter insertion site

Rationale:

Correct answer: C, D

A suprapubic catheter is surgically placed into the bladder through an abdominal incision with a dressing over the site. The insertion site should be assessed every eight hours for signs of infection including erythema, swelling, tenderness, and drainage. When cleaning the insertion site, the nurse should gently pull on the catheter to help loosen any debris that has become encrusted between the skin and the catheter.

A is incorrect because sterile technique does not need to be used to care for the suprapubic catheter. Aseptic technique is used when cleaning the suprapubic catheter insertion site with half-strength hydrogen peroxide and sterile water in a medicine cup with clean gloves and a sterile cotton ball. A circular motion is used to remove debris, but the area should not be scrubbed vigorously. The nurse should wipe in a circular motion starting at the insertion site and moving outwards.

B is incorrect because wiping toward the insertion site is not aseptic technique and increases risk for infection.

E is incorrect because the balloon should not be deflated during cleaning or dressing changes. The balloon is deflated when the catheter is to be removed.

93. The nurse is preparing to insert a nasogastric tube in a patient on the medical-surgical floor. The nurse knows nasogastric tubes can be utilized for which of the following? (Select all that apply):

  A. Gastric decompression
  B. Instilling of medications
  C. Parenteral feeding
  D. Banding of esophageal varices
  E. Evaluation of gastrointestinal bleeding

Rationale:

Correct answer: A, B, E

The indications for nasogastric tubes include gastric decompression or suctioning out of gastric contents, instilling of medications, enteral feeding, and evaluation of gastrointestinal bleeding.

C is incorrect because nasogastric tubes are used for enteral feedings, not parenteral feeding.

D is incorrect because nasogastric tubes are contraindicated in esophageal varices banding as the NG insertion procedure can cause trauma and bleeding.

94. The nurse is caring for five patients on the medical-surgical floor and needs to delegate care to the unlicensed assistive personnel (UAP). Which of the following can the nurse delegate to the UAP? (Select all that apply):

  A. Administration of an enema to a comatose patient
  B. Removing a fecal impaction from a patient on bed rest after a spinal injury
  C. Putting a patient on the bedpan after hip replacement surgery
  D. Insertion of a nasogastric tube to a patient with a cerebral aneurysm
  E. Providing oral care to a patient with nasogastric tube

Rationale:

Correct answer: A, C, E

It is within the unlicensed assistive personnel's scope of practice to administer an enema, put a patient on the bedpan, and provide oral care.

Note: UAP can perform a task if it routinely occurs in the care of patients, is performed according to an established set of steps, involves little or no modification from one patient-care situation to another, may be performed with a predictable outcome, does not inherently involve ongoing assessment, interpretation, or decision-making, and does not endanger a client's life or well-being.

B is incorrect because removal of fecal impactions can cause stimulation of the vagus nerve and bradycardia, so this is the nurse's responsibility because the task requires ongoing assessment.

D is incorrect because insertion of a nasogastric tube risks aspiration and is the nurse's responsibility. Additionally, a patient with a cerebral aneurysm needs to be monitored for increases in ICP, especially during procedures, so this requires the nurse's assessment.

95. The nurse is caring for a 67-year-old patient who has a urinary diversion in place. When the nurse inserts a catheter into the diversion to obtain a urine sample, only a scant amount of urine is returned to the drainage bag. In order to obtain a larger sample which action should be performed by the nurse first? (Select all that apply):

    A. Remove the catheter and use the pouch for the sample
    B. Advance the catheter into the urinary diversion
    C. Apply gentle pressure to the patient's abdomen
    D. Turn the patient on their side
    E. Use a needle and sterile technique to withdraw a urine sample directly from the bladder

Rationale:

Correct answer: B, C, D

Advancing the catheter, massaging the abdomen, and repositioning the patient can all be attempted by the nurse in order to obtain a more adequate sample.

A is incorrect because the urine in the pouch is contaminated. The urine sample must be obtained directly from the diversion catheter or the bladder.

E is incorrect because it is not within the nurse's scope of practice to insert a needle through the abdominal wall into the bladder. This risks infection and bladder rupture.

96. A patient on the oncology unit is one day post-op from urostomy creation due to cancer of the genitourinary tract. Which of the following behaviors by the patient demonstrate acceptance of bodily function alteration? (Select all that apply):

    A. The patient watches the nurse change the pouch
    B. The patient asks the nurse about how the urostomy works
    C. The patient empties the pouch themselves
    D. The patient assures the nurse their spouse will change the pouch at home

E. The patient focuses on the television while the nurse is changing the pouch.

Rationale:

Correct answer: A, B, C

If the patient accepts the change in body function, observing the nurse perform the procedure is a positive sign of readiness to learn. Asking questions demonstrates active participation in the care of the urostomy and indicates acceptance of the urinary diversion. Performing the procedure themselves is the ultimate goal, which signifies the patient is not in denial and has accepted the change, and is willing to provide self-care.

D is incorrect because it demonstrates avoidance of self-care, which is a component of denial.

E is incorrect because this shows lack of interest. The nurse should be sure that the TV is off and all other distractions are minimized when teaching or demonstrating care.

97. A patient with a new urostomy is in the clinic for follow-up. Which of the following symptoms would cause the nurse to suspect a urinary tract infection (UTI)? (Select all that apply):

    A. Difficulty recalling their spouse's name
    B. Upper abdominal pain
    C. Dark, concentrated urine
    D. Foul-smelling urine
    E. Urine output 800 mL in six hours

Rationale:

Correct answer: A, C, D

A UTI is commonly characterized by dark or even bloody, as well as foul-smelling urine, fever, confusion, and flank pain. (Note: the elderly may not show increased temperature with presence of a UTI due to decreased ability for thermoregulation as a part of the natural aging process.)

B is incorrect because pain from a UTI is usually localized to the flank on the posterior side of the body. The organs of the urinary tract are found in the lower abdomen, not the upper abdomen.

E is incorrect because a UTI does not cause increased urine output. This patient has put out over 100 mL of urine per hour for the last six hours, which is abnormally high. The patient may be at risk for dehydration due to over-diuresis, and the healthcare provider should be notified, but a UTI will not be suspected.

98. Prevention of surgical site infections requires collaboration of the surgical team, nursing team, and the patient and family. Which of the following measures are used to prevent surgical site infections? (Select all that apply):

    A. Discharge the patient as soon as possible
    B. Shampoo the patient's hair before neck or back surgery
    C. Administration of PO prophylactic antibiotic within an hour of the incision
    D. Shave surgical sites carefully with a razor before surgery
    E. Control blood sugar levels in diabetic as well as nondiabetic patients
    F. Have the patient shower before preoperative enema is excreted

Rationale:

Correct answer: A, B, E

All of the interventions are indicated for reduction of surgical site infections. Longer hospital stays are associated with hospital-acquired infections, so discharge as soon as possible is beneficial. Neck and back surgery may prevent the patient from properly washing their hair for up to a week afterward, so starting with a clean head is important to reduce bacteria that may remain in the hair or on the scalp postoperatively. An abnormal increase or decrease in blood sugars can increase risk for infection.

C is incorrect because prophylactic antibiotics are given IV shortly before surgery. The patient should not be given anything by mouth within an hour of the surgical incision. Generally, patients are NPO for eight hours pre-operatively.

D is incorrect because shaving with a razor can create microvascular cuts, which increases risk for infection. Clippers are now used for hair removal before surgery.

F is incorrect because thoroughly cleaning the body *after* a pre-operative enema will reduce the bacteria that enters the OR on the patient's body.

99. The nurse in the medical-surgical unit notes 50 mL of bright red drainage in a patient's Jackson-Pratt (JP) drain four hours after breast reconstruction surgery. Which of the following interventions should the nurse perform? (Select all that apply):

    A. Empty the drain in 24 hours
    B. Pin the tubing to the patient's gown
    C. Place Vaseline gauze around the insertion site
    D. Secure the drain above the wound
    E. Empty the drain
    F. Squeeze the JP flat and plug it

Rationale:

Correct answer: B, E, F

A JP drain is used in wound care to collect exudate, measure it, protect the surrounding skin, contain micro-organisms, and reduce the frequency of care. JP drains are put in place during a surgical procedure, with subsequent nursing care until they are removed. No external suction is necessary as the bulb is squeezed flat and plugged, which naturally applies suction. The drain should be pinned to the patient's gown below the level of the insertion site. This drain should be emptied, measured, then squeezed flat to continue draining the cavity. Documentation for drains includes the amount of drainage, its appearance and odor, and the assessment findings for the surrounding skin.

A is incorrect because the JP drain should be monitored for drainage frequently according to facility policy. The drain should be emptied when full, when inflated (indicating need for compression), and per shift.

C is incorrect because the site does not require Vaseline gauze but a sterile cotton dressing.

D is incorrect because the JP drain is secured to the patient's gown *below* the level of insertion site to prevent backflow of drainage into the site.

100. The nurse is preparing to irrigate a patient's wound. Which of the following are acceptable interventions for irrigating a wound? (Select all that apply):

    A. Introduce the irrigation solution by allowing it to run from the top of the wound to the bottom of the wound where it is absorbed into a pad beneath the wound
    B. Mechanical cleansing with sterile solution and instruments
    C. Apply antibiotic ointment to the wound edges before irrigating
    D. Chill the irrigation solution to 65°F or just below room temperature
    E. Pre-medicate with analgesics

Rationale:

Correct answer: A, B, E

Passive irrigation (as described in A) involves solution and gravity. This allows microorganisms, loose tissue, and debris to run down and away from the wound gradually. Debridement is the use of sterile instruments to mechanically cleanse a wound with sterile solution and gauze and is another effective way to cleanse a wound and remove debris.

When irrigating a wound, sterile technique and directing solution from healthy to infected tissue reduces risk of infection. Wound irrigation is used to clean out drainage, foreign material, and microorganisms that contribute to infection. The wound irrigation procedure can be painful, so assessing and pre-treating pain is beneficial and will help the patient tolerate the procedure.

C is incorrect because if any ointment is to be used, it should be applied after the irrigation procedure is complete and the wound edges have been dried.

D is incorrect because irrigation solution should be at room temperature to reduce discomfort during the procedure.

CHAPTER 3:

NCLEX-RN – FUNDAMENTALS: SAFETY/INFECTION CONTROL

Multiple Choice

1. The nurse finds a patient unresponsive on the floor and isn't sure if the patient has a head injury from a fall. What is the first action the nurse should perform to prevent the patient from being injured further?

    A. Perform a head-to-toe assessment
    B. Apply a cervical collar
    C. Call for assistance to return the patient to bed
    D. Notify the healthcare provider

    Rationale:

    Correct answer: B

    Any time a head or neck injury is suspected, a cervical collar should be applied. This is the only choice that prevents further injury to the patient.

    A is incorrect because an assessment will not prevent further injury to the patient. The cervical collar must be applied before the nurse performs a thorough assessment.

    C is incorrect because using additional people to return the patient to bed will not prevent injury to the patient. The patient should remain where found, and the nurse should assess for injury before moving them.

    D is incorrect because notifying the healthcare provider will not prevent further injury to the patient. The nurse should focus on the patient, apply a C-collar, assess for airway, breathing, and circulation to determine how to intervene next.

2. A patient on the medical-surgical unit calls the nurse to report a fire in the trash can. Which of the following actions by the nurse is inappropriate?

A. Turn off oxygen to the room

B. Evacuate the patient from the room

C. Call for help

D. Have the patient throw a blanket over the trash can

Rationale:

Correct answer: D

The proper response to a fire is RACE: Rescue, Alert, Contain, Evacuate. Having the patient throw a blanket over a fire in a trash can is an inappropriate action by the nurse. The blanket will contain the fire but containment is not to be done until the patient has been rescued from the area and the fire alarm has been pulled.

A is incorrect because turning off oxygen to a room where there is a fire is an appropriate action.

B is incorrect because evacuating the patient from the room is an appropriate action.

C is incorrect because calling for help is an appropriate action.

3. The nurse on the cardiac intensive care unit is caring for an unstable patient post cardiac surgery. The patient remains orally intubated on the ventilator, as weaning has failed. Which of the following solutions could decrease the risk of ventilator-assisted pneumonia (VAP) in this intubated patient?

A. Peroxide

B. Normal saline

C. Chlorhexidine

D. Toothbrushing with fluoridated tap water

Rationale:

Correct answer: C

The prevalence of hospital-acquired infection is a significant concern in acutely and critically ill patients. Ventilator-associated pneumonia (VAP) contributes to mortality in critically ill patients. Studies have shown chlorhexidine to be effective and safe in intubated patients to prevent VAP as it kills bacteria.

VAP occurs in patients who are intubated and on the ventilator for more than 24-48 hours and is prevented through the use of chlorhexidine oral solution for frequent oral care, frequent handwashing, raising the head of the bed at least 45 degrees, and frequent suctioning. If a feeding tube is needed, it is important to place the end of the tube beyond the pylorus of the stomach to reduce VAP.

A is incorrect because peroxide is not recommended for oral care in ventilated patients. Half-strength hydrogen peroxide may be used to provide tracheostomy care, but this patient does not have a tracheostomy in place.

B is incorrect because normal saline does not prevent VAP.

D is incorrect because neither tap water nor fluoride prevents VAP. It is difficult to brush the teeth of a patient with an oral endotracheal tube in place so soft swabs are used instead.

4. The nurse on the cardiac unit finds a patient unresponsive in a bathroom. What is the first action the nurse should perform?

   A. Start chest compressions
   B. Check for a pulse
   C. Call for help
   D. Get an automated external defibrillator (AED)

Rationale:

Correct answer: C

Upon finding a patient unresponsive, the first action should be to call for help. This will mobilize people to assist with resuscitative efforts as applicable, as well as bring necessary equipment, such as an AED.

A is incorrect because chest compressions should not be started until lack of a pulse has been confirmed and the nurse has called for assistance.

B is incorrect because checking the patient for a pulse should be done immediately after calling for help.

D is incorrect because the AED should be brought by another staff member when the nurse calls for help. The nurse should not leave the patient alone on the floor to obtain equipment.

5. A patient is experiencing dysphagia after a stroke. Which of the following foods should the nurse offer the patient?

   A. Applesauce
   B. Shredded wheat and milk
   C. Jell-O

D. Lemon sherbet

Rationale:

Correct answer: A

Patients experiencing dysphagia are at risk for aspiration and have an easier time swallowing single textures. Thin liquids and multiple textures put the patient at risk of aspirating their meal. Measures that facilitate swallowing include sitting the client upright with their neck flexed slightly, instructing the patient to use tongue actively, placing food on the unaffected side of the mouth, and maintaining an upright position 30-45 minutes after eating.

B is incorrect because shredded wheat and milk have multiple textures. Milk products should be avoided in the patient with dysphagia because these products can cause saliva to become thick and sticky.

C is incorrect because Jell-O is a thin liquid.

D is incorrect because sherbet is a thin liquid.

6. The nurse is caring for patients on the rehabilitation unit who are receiving open system enteral feedings. The nurse knows the most important intervention for preventing infections related to enteral feedings is:

   A. Use sterile technique to insert nasogastric tubes
   B. Keep enteral feeding solutions cold
   C. Handle the feeding system using aseptic technique
   D. Changing tubing with each feeding

Rationale:

Correct answer: C

Enteral feeding solutions can grow bacteria; therefore, it is important to use aseptic technique when handling the feeding system, formula, and tubing connections. An open system requires the nurse to open a can of feeding solution and pour it into a bag that infuses through tubing into the patient's feeding tube. The solution should not stand for more than four hours.

A is incorrect because insertion of a nasogastric tube does not require sterile technique. This is a clean procedure.

B is incorrect because keeping the enteral feeding cold will not prevent bacteria from growing if contaminated. Enteral feeding should be administered at room temperature to prevent discomfort.

D is incorrect because tubing should be changed every 24 hours and irrigated after every feeding and once per shift to maintain patency.

7. A 74-year-old man is in the hospital after surgery. When assessing for postoperative infection, which is the priority assessment by the nurse?

    A. Change in behavior
    B. Daily white blood cell count
    C. Presence of fever and chills
    D. Tolerance of increasing activity

Rationale:

Correct answer: A

Immune function decreases in older patients and may not demonstrate classic infection signs including increased white blood cells, fever, or localized signs. Change in behavior or mental status may be the only (or the earliest) sign of infection in older patients.

B is incorrect because white blood cell count may be normal in an elderly client with an infection present due to the natural aging process and its effect on the immune system.

C is incorrect because presence of fever and chills is not indicative of infection by itself. These symptoms may not be present in an elderly patient.

D is incorrect because while tolerance of increasing activity is a good outcome, is not indicative of infection.

8. A patient is being prepared for discharge home after surgery. A large dressing will need to be changed and a drain managed by the patient. What is the most important instruction by the nurse?

    A. "Be sure you keep all your postoperative appointments."
    B. "Call your surgeon if you have any questions at home."
    C. "Eat a diet high in protein, iron, zinc, and vitamin C."
    D. "Wash your hands before touching the drain or dressing."

Rationale:

Correct answer: D

All options are appropriate for the client being discharged after surgery. However, for this client who is changing a dressing and managing a drain, infection prevention is the greatest priority. The nurse should instruct the client to wash their hands often, including before and after touching the dressing or drain.

A is incorrect because keeping postoperative appointments does not confirm ability of the patient to care for the dressing and drain. Addressing post-op infection is highest priority.

B is incorrect because calling the surgeon may be appropriate but does not confirm ability of the patient to care for the dressing and drain.

C is incorrect because diet does not confirm ability of the patient to care for the dressing and drain and does not promote infection prevention. Protein, zinc, and vitamin C can help promote wound healing. Protein also provides energy for cell growth and iron helps prevent anemia. (Zinc supplementation is sometimes used to prevent colds but has not been proven effective.)

9. A patient is scheduled for magnetic resonance imaging (MRI) of their heart. The patient's medical history includes a myocardial infarction and permanent pacemaker. Which of the following actions should the nurse take?

    A. Schedule an electrocardiogram just before the MRI
    B. Notify the healthcare provider before scheduling the MRI
    C. Call the physician and request a laboratory draw for cardiac enzymes
    D. Instruct the patient to increase fluid intake the day before the MRI

Rationale:

Correct answer: A

The current guidelines from the American Heart Association and the Food and Drug Administration (FDA) do not support MRI use in pacemaker patients. The magnetic field of the MRI can deactivate or damage the pacemaker or rapid pacing may be triggered. Other adverse outcomes may include inappropriate shocks or burning the skin over the pacemaker implantation site. The healthcare provider should be notified of the patient's pacemaker so another diagnostic test can be ordered. MRI is only used with patients who have pacemakers when other alternative radiologic tests have been unsuccessful in making a diagnosis.

A is incorrect because an electrocardiogram is not needed.

C is incorrect because the patient does not need cardiac enzymes. These would be drawn if the nurse suspects an MI now but not required simply due to a past history of MI.

D is incorrect because increased fluids are not needed.

10. A patient just underwent lung biopsy and is in the recovery period. Which finding by the nurse would require immediate action?

    A. Increased temperature
    B. Absent breath sounds
    C. Productive cough
    D. Incisional discomfort

Rationale:

Correct answer: B

Absent breath sounds may indicate a pneumothorax, a serious complication after needle biopsy or open lung biopsy. Pneumothorax is a condition in which air enters the pleural space and causes the affected lung to have less expansion room and potentially may even collapse.

A is incorrect because increased temperature is not life-threatening but may be a sign of infection. Infection from lung biopsy would not present with elevated temperature immediately after the procedure.

C is incorrect because a productive cough is not life-threatening.

D is incorrect because incisional discomfort is expected and is not life-threatening.

11. The student nurse is caring for a patient with a tracheostomy. During the procedure, which student action would require the instructor to intervene?

    A. Holding the device securely when changing ties
    B. Suctioning the patient's mouth after trach care is complete
    C. Applying suction for 20-30 seconds while withdrawing the catheter
    D. Using half-strength peroxide for cleansing

Rationale:

Correct answer: C

Suction should be applied for no more than 10-15 seconds while withdrawing the catheter. If the student nurse suctions for too long, this can cause hypoxia. Suctioning should be limited to three times, and the patient should be hyperoxygenated in between suction passes.

A is incorrect because holding the device when changing ties is appropriate. This prevents the tracheostomy tube from becoming displaced, so no intervention is required.

B is incorrect because it is appropriate to provide oral care after tracheostomy care is completed, so no intervention is required.

D is incorrect because half-strength peroxide is indicated for cleaning during trach care and rinsing the inner cannula. No intervention is necessary.

12. The nurse is teaching at the community health center about how to prevent lower back injuries and pain. Which of the following instructions should be included by the nurse?

    A. "Participate in an exercise program to strengthen muscles."
    B. "Purchase a mattress that allows you to adjust the firmness."
    C. "Wear flat instead of high-heeled shoes to work each day."
    D. "Keep your weight within 20% of your ideal body weight."

Rationale:

Correct answer: A

A common myth is that exercise should be avoided when a patient experiences back pain. Exercise has the ability to strengthen back and core muscles, which can reduce and even prevent incidence of lower back pain. Stretching can also increase range of motion, preventing back pain. Patients should also be taught safe work practices such as avoiding awkward posture, preventing over-exertion, and limiting repetitive activities and fatigue.

B is incorrect because a mattress may not prevent lower back pain and it is unrealistic to assume the patient has the means to purchase a new mattress. The nurse must suggest realistic interventions that are most likely to achieve results.

C is incorrect because wearing flats may not prevent lower back pain.

D is incorrect because maintaining weight alone may not prevent lower back.

13. A patient who underwent spinal fusion is being prepared for discharge. When providing postoperative instructions to the patient, which statement should be included by the nurse?

    A. "Only lift items that are 10 pounds or less."
    B. "Wear your brace whenever you are out of bed."
    C. "Remain in bed for three days after surgery, and then gradually increase your activity."
    D. "You are prescribed medications to prevent rejection."

Rationale:

Correct answer: B

Spinal fusion is performed to repair and remove bone and tissue that narrows the spinal canal, causing squeezing of the cord and pain. Patients who undergo spinal fusion are fitted for a brace that must be worn for 3-6 months, throughout the healing process, anytime the patient is out of bed.

A is incorrect because these patients should not lift anything initially when going home after spinal fusion surgery.

C is incorrect because the patient will not be discharged home until they can successfully get out of bed. Mobility is an important component of the recovery from spinal fusion surgery as it increases quality of life and helps prevent complications such as pneumonia and blood clot formation.

D is incorrect because anti-rejection medication is not prescribed for this procedure. After spinal fusion, the nurse would expect the patient to be prescribed analgesics and antispasmodics.

14. A nursing instructor is teaching students about infection control. Which of the following is the most effective barrier for infection prevention?

    A. Colonization by host bacteria
    B. Gastrointestinal secretions
    C. Inflammatory processes
    D. Skin and mucous membranes

Rationale:

Correct answer: D

The most important barriers against infection are the skin and mucous membranes.

A is incorrect because colonization by host bacteria is a barrier but not the most effective. Each person has their own normal flora, which are healthy bacteria that compete with foreign pathogens for attachment sites to body cells.

B is incorrect because GI secretions are a barrier but not the most effective. GI secretions are acidic in nature, killing many forms of bacteria that may enter the stomach.

C is incorrect because the inflammatory process is a barrier but not the most effective. The inflammatory process involves migration of the body's white blood cells to an area of infection and killing the foreign bacteria before they have the chance to multiply.

15. A nurse unit manager has noticed an upward trend in infection rates in the unit. Which of the following actions would help the manager in determining how to best prevent infection on the unit?

A. Auditing staff members' hand hygiene practices

B. Ensuring clients are placed in appropriate isolation

C. Establishing a policy to remove urinary catheters quickly

D. Teaching staff members about infection control methods

Rationale:

Correct answer: A

Poor hand hygiene in healthcare workers is the biggest cause of hospital-acquired infections. Clean hands are the single most important factor in preventing the spread of pathogens. A hand hygiene audit can be performed by the manager or designee to find out if poor hand hygiene is a cause of the increased rate of infections on the unit. A hand hygiene audit assesses for frequency of hand cleaning, use of soap or alcohol–based rub, type of soap used, time hands were scrubbed, whether all surfaces of hands were washed, method of drying, and use of a pedal trash bin.

B is incorrect because appropriate isolation practices can help prevent spread of infection from patient to patient, or from patient to healthcare worker, but it is not a primary method for preventing infection from occurring.

C is incorrect because removal of urinary catheters can prevent catheter-associated urinary tract infections (CAUTI) but it is not a primary method for preventing infection.

D is incorrect because teaching healthcare workers about infection control methods is important, but this does not give the nurse manager any information about how to prevent infection on the unit.

16. A student nurse is caring for patients on the intensive care unit nurse. When the student asks what role tooth brushing has in infection control, what is the best response by the registered nurse?

A. "Brushing teeth helps to remove biofilm, which can spread microorganisms."

B. "The toothbrush helps to clean all surfaces."

C. "Oral care is important to all our patients."

D. "Toothbrushes last longer than oral swabs and can be cleaned easier."

Rationale:

Correct answer: A

Biofilms are bacteria in complex groups within gel which can accumulate on surfaces like the teeth. Dental plaque biofilms are responsible for many of the diseases that commonly cause dental caries and other oral infections. Disruption is the most effective way to control biofilms, such as is achieved by tooth-brushing.

B is incorrect because it is not accurate. Proper technique is needed to reach most surfaces of the teeth with a toothbrush but one cannot assume that all surfaces are reached.

C is incorrect because it does not answer the student's question.

D is incorrect because it is inaccurate and does not address the spread of infection.

17. A patient is admitted to the emergency room with possible sepsis. Which of the following is highest priority for this patient?

    A. Antibiotic administration
    B. Antipyretic administration
    C. Obtain blood cultures
    D. Place the patient in isolation

Rationale:

Correct answer: C

Blood cultures (or urine, sputum, etc.) are the priority to collect on a patient suspected to have sepsis. This must be performed before broad-spectrum antibiotics are initiated. The results of the cultures may take several days, so the antibiotics will be started after the cultures have been collected.

A is incorrect because administering antibiotics before cultures are collected will affect results.

B is incorrect because antipyretics are given for fever, which may be associated with sepsis, but blood cultures are the highest priority.

D is incorrect because isolation may not be needed, depending on the source and type of infection.

18. A patient on the medical-surgical floor is receiving several antibiotics and develops frequent watery stools. What is the most important action by the nurse?

    A. Obtain stool cultures
    B. Ensure that the client has frequent perianal care
    C. Do not allow the client to have anything by mouth until the diarrhea resolves
    D. Request a prescription for an anti-diarrheal medication

Rationale:

Correct answer: A

Clostridium difficile is suspected in admitted patient experiencing three or more stools per day for two days or more. The healthcare provider should be notified and the nurse should obtain stool cultures.

B is incorrect because perianal care is important for preventing skin breakdown in a patient experiencing frequent watery stool but is not the priority.

C is incorrect because the NPO status is not required for a patient with *Clostridium difficile*. The nurse must ensure adequate fluids to prevent dehydration, as the patient is losing water through the diarrhea.

D is incorrect because anti-diarrheal medication stops the diarrhea and prevents the bacteria from exiting the body.

19. The unlicensed assistive personnel (UAP) is performing hygiene and changing bed sheets for a patient under the observation of a nurse. What action by the UAP requires intervention by the nurse?

    A. Combing the patient's hair while wearing gloves
    B. Rinsing the patient's commode pan after use
    C. Gently shaking dirty linens and placing them on the floor
    D. Using gloves when providing perianal care

Rationale:

Correct answer: C

Shaking clean or dirty linens can spread microbes through the air. Placing linens on the floor leads to spread of infection via healthcare workers' shoes.

A is incorrect because C is a greater concern. It is unnecessary to wear gloves when caring for a patient's hair unless a scalp infection is present. (It is not harmful to wear gloves, though.)

B is incorrect because it is appropriate to rinse a commode pan after use.

D is incorrect because it is appropriate to wear gloves during perianal care.

20. A bioterrorism drill is performed in the medical-surgical unit. The nursing team is preparing to admit a patient with inhalation anthrax. Which type of precautions should the nursing team prepare for?

    A. Airborne precautions
    B. Contact precautions
    C. Droplet precautions
    D. Standard precautions

Rationale:

Correct answer: D

Bioterrorism is the intentional release of viruses, bacteria, or other germs that can sicken or kill people, livestock, or crops. *Bacillus anthracis*, the bacteria that causes anthrax, is one of the most likely agents to be used in a biological attack. Symptoms include fever, chills, chest discomfort, shortness of breath, confusion or dizziness, cough, drenching sweats, nausea, vomiting, headache, and body aches.

If untreated, all types of anthrax have the potential to spread throughout the body and cause severe illness and even death. Standard precautions are needed for a patient admitted with anthrax inhalation. Inhaled anthrax is not spread from person to person.

A is incorrect because airborne precautions are not necessary.

B is incorrect because contact precautions are not necessary.

C is incorrect because droplet precautions are not necessary.

21. The nurse is caring for four patients on the medical-surgical unit. How does the nurse help prevent these patients from contracting a hospital-acquired infection?

   A. Assess skin and mucous membranes
   B. Use appropriate hand hygiene consistently
   C. Assess white blood cell counts frequently
   D. Keep visitors away when they are ill

Rationale:

Correct answer: B

Hand hygiene is the number one way to prevent infection because most healthcare-associated infections are caused by contaminated healthcare workers' hands.

A is incorrect because assessing skin and mucous membranes can help the nurse identify infection quickly but not prevent it.

C is incorrect because monitoring lab results will help the nurse identify infection quickly but not prevent it.

D is incorrect because it can prevent infection, but not as much as consistent hand hygiene.

22. The medical unit nurse admits a patient with a fever, papular rash on the face, palms, and soles of the feet, and generalized muscle pain. What is the first action the nurse should take?

    A. Culture the lesions
    B. Place the patient on airborne precautions isolation
    C. Ensure that antibiotics are administered as ordered
    D. Provide comfort measures for the rash

Rationale:

Correct answer: B

This patient has the signs and symptoms of smallpox infection. A single case is a public health emergency. This patient should be placed on airborne, contact, and standard precautions before any other interventions are performed. Smallpox symptoms (fever, myalgia, rash) occur within 7-10 days of exposure. The rash scabs over within 1-2 weeks, and the patient is contagious until the scabs separate in about three weeks.

A is incorrect because cultures are not the first action to be taken.

C is incorrect because antibiotics are not the first action to be taken.

D is incorrect because other physical needs are a greater priority than comfort measures.

23. The family of a patient under contact precautions is fearful of visiting and becoming infected by the patient. What is the best action by the nurse?

    A. Inform the family that these precautions are mandated by law
    B. Reassure the family that they cannot get the infection
    C. Inform the family that if contact precautions are followed, it is unlikely that the disease will be spread to healthcare workers or visitors
    D. Tell the family it is important for the patient's wellbeing that they visit the patient

Rationale:

Correct answer: C

Isolation precautions can have a negative effect on families and patients. The nurse should explain the purpose of contact precautions and inform the family of what is being done to treat the patient. The nurse should help the family make a decision that they are comfortable with.

A is incorrect because it does not address the family's concerns or help the family make a decision about visiting the patient.

B is incorrect because it offers false reassurance. The family must make a decision about visiting the patient, knowing that if precautions aren't followed, a chance of infection exists.

D is incorrect because this statement may make the family feel obligated to come and visit. The nurse should give factual information to help the family make a decision about visiting the patient.

24. The nurse is caring for a patient diagnosed with a urinary tract infection (UTI) caused by methicillin-resistant *Staphylococcus aureus* (MRSA). What is the most appropriate action by the nurse?

    A. Administer vancomycin
    B. Limit visitors to immediate family only
    C. Wash hands only after taking off gloves after care
    D. Use a respirator mask when measuring and disposing of urine

Rationale:

Correct answer: A

Vancomycin is approved for use in treating MRSA. MRSA is an antibiotic-resistant infection that can spread easily if infection precautions are not followed specifically.

B is incorrect because visitation does not need to be limited.

C is incorrect because hand hygiene should be performed both before and after wearing gloves.

D is incorrect because airborne precautions are not necessary, although a face shield should be utilized because splashing may occur when handling bodily fluids of any patient, not only patients with MRSA.

25. A patient admitted under contact precautions has a computed tomography (CT) scan ordered. What is the most appropriate action by the nurse?

    A. Ensure that the radiology department is aware of the isolation precautions
    B. Make arrangements to go with the patient to ensure appropriate precautions are used
    C. Send the patient for the CT and resume contact precautions when the patient returns from the procedure
    D. Notify the physician that the patient cannot leave the room for the CT scan

Rationale:

Correct answer: A

Patients who are admitted under contract precautions should only leave their rooms for necessary purposes, such as CT scans or other medical procedures. The radiology department needs to be made aware of the isolation precautions needed for this patient.

(Note: If a similar patient needs physical therapy (PT), for example, it is not safe to transfer them to the physical therapy department where they may increase risk for infections of others. The PT would be encouraged to come to the patient's room for PT while the patient is on contact precautions.)

B is incorrect because the nurse only needs to go with the patient if the patient is unstable or needs cardiac monitoring.

C is incorrect because contact precautions must be maintained while transferring the patient and while in the CT procedure room.

D is incorrect because the patient can leave for CT but contact precautions must be maintained. It is unsafe to delay the diagnostic procedure.

26. A patient in the clinic has an infected wound on the right upper extremity. What can the nurse delegate to the unlicensed assistive personnel (UAP) as a comfort measure?

    A. Order a fan to help cool the patient if feverish
    B. Place cool, wet compresses on top of the wound
    C. Place the arm above the level of the heart
    D. Take the patient's temperature every four hours

Rationale:

Correct answer: C

Elevating the arm will help decrease swelling and pain. This can be delegated to the UAP.

A is incorrect because a fan can spread microbes throughout the room, increasing transmission of disease to other patient or healthcare workers.

B is incorrect because a cool, wet compress can macerate broken skin.

D is incorrect because checking temperature is not a comfort measure.

27. Laboratory reports for a patient admitted with a fever indicate a shift to the left in the white blood cell count. What is the most important action by the nurse?

    A. Make notation of the findings and continue to monitor the client
    B. Call the healthcare provider with the expectation of an antibiotics order
    C. Tell the UAP to place the patient in protective isolation

D. Tell the patient this signifies inflammation

Rationale:

Correct answer: B

A shift to the left in a white blood cell count indicates immature neutrophil increase. As a part of the inflammatory response, the bone marrow releases immature WBCs into the bloodstream. This is indicative of bacterial infection. The healthcare provider should be notified of an antibiotic order.

A is incorrect because continued monitoring does not address the potential infection.

C is incorrect because isolation is not appropriate until a culture deems it necessary.

D is incorrect because teaching should be done but it is not the most important action. Physical care of the patient takes priority over patient education.

28. A patient is admitted to the emergency with suspected bacterial meningitis. The nurse administers antibiotics for the virus as directed by the healthcare provider. Which of the following is the most appropriate action the nurse should perform?

    A. Assess the client frequently for neurological decline.
    B. Tell the unlicensed assistive personnel to be sure to keep client comfortable.
    C. Ensure the client is placed on Contact Precautions.
    D. Limit visitors to the immediate family only.

Rationale:

Correct answer: A

Meningitis is an infection of the meninges that line the inside of the brain and spinal column. It can be caused by bacteria, virus, or fungus. The nurse needs to monitor the patient's neurological status frequently for worsening of the condition.

B is incorrect because comfort measures are appropriate for any patient but not more important than physical care of the patient.

C is incorrect because patients with suspected meningitis are placed on droplet precautions upon admission. Gown, gloves, masks, and goggles must be worn by anyone coming into close contact with the patient.

D is incorrect because visitation does not need to be restricted. The nurse is responsible for educating the visitors about the use of personal protective equipment if they are to come into close contact with the patient.

29. The nurse is caring for a patient with chronic myeloid leukemia. When the patient asks the nurse why they are still at increased risk for infection since their white blood cell count (WBC) is elevated, what is the best response by the nurse?

    A. "Your WBCs are high, which means you already have an infection."
    B. "Leukemia means your body is in a blast crisis with too many WBCs."
    C. "Your lab results must be a mistake; your WBCs should be very low."
    D. "Your WBCs are abnormal and cannot provide protection against infection."

Rationale:

Correct answer: D

The WBCs in leukemia are abnormal and do not have the ability to provide protection against infection.

A is incorrect because it is an inaccurate statement.

B is incorrect because it is an inaccurate statement. Myeloid leukemia is divided into three phases: chronic, accelerated, or blast phase. This patient is in the chronic phase when the blood and bone marrow contain 10-19% blast cells (immature WBCs). Blast phase is characterized by more than 20% blast cells.

C is incorrect because it is an inaccurate statement and does not address the risk for infection.

30. A patient is admitted to the emergency room with symptoms of tuberculosis (TB). What is the most important action the nurse needs to perform?

    A. Administer normal saline by IV
    B. Apply a nasal cannula and administer oxygen
    C. Obtain a sputum culture
    D. Place the patient in a negative pressure room

Rationale:

Correct answer: D

Any patient with symptoms of tuberculosis or airborne pathogens must first be placed in a negative pressure room to prevent spread of infection. Due to the highly contagious nature of TB, isolation is the nurse's greatest priority before providing any other patient care. This is for the safety of the nurse, the healthcare team, and the other patients.

A is incorrect because IV fluids are not the most important action.

B is incorrect because oxygen is not indicated unless the patient has low oxygen saturation or shows signs of hypoxia. Isolation still takes priority over oxygen, even if oxygen is needed.

C is incorrect because a sputum culture is not the most important action.

31. The emergency room nurse is assessing a patient who is unresponsive and wearing an oxygen mask. What is the most important action the nurse should perform first?

    A. Assess neurologic status
    B. Determine if the patient's breathing is adequate
    C. Start a large bore IV
    D. Place the patient on the cardiac monitor

Rationale:

Correct answer: B

Breathing is the highest priority for the unresponsive patient and must be assessed by the nurse. If the patient has a mask on and is not breathing, the oxygen running through the mask is not effectively reaching the lungs. The nurse must first determine if rescue breaths need to be administered immediately.

A is incorrect because neurologic assessment will be performed after the nurse assesses and ensures adequate breathing and circulation.

C is incorrect because starting an IV to administer fluids is not more important than assessing breathing.

D is incorrect because placing the patient on the cardiac monitor will not give the nurse information about breathing status.

32. The nurse has taught a community water safety class at the city center. Which of the following statements by a client indicates the nurse needs to provide more education?

    A. "I can swim by myself, now."
    B. "My toddler cannot be left alone in the bathtub, even for a short period of time."
    C. "Any time I have a pool party, an adult should supervise the pool."
    D. "In case of an emergency, I will keep a phone near my pool."

Rationale:

Correct answer: A

Whether or not a person has lifeguard status, people should not swim alone. If an emergency occurs and a person is alone, emergency response can be delayed.

B is incorrect because it indicates good understanding. Toddlers can drown in even a small amount of water. They are not able to make mature decisions about their safety and should be supervised in the bathtub at all times.

C is incorrect because it indicates good understanding. Children should not be left unattended, even for brief periods of time, while in or near a pool.

D is incorrect because it indicates good understanding. A working phone should be available near the pool so someone can call for help if needed. This is a safe action that is encouraged in water safety education.

33. The nurse is caring for a patient who sustained an acute burn injury. Which action by the nurse can prevent auto-contamination infection when caring for the burn?

    A. Advocate for consistent handwashing by the healthcare staff
    B. Change gloves when caring for wounds on different parts of the patient's body
    C. Use a disposable blood pressure cuff instead of sharing with other patients
    D. Use a closed method of burn management for wound care

Rationale:

Correct answer: B

Auto contamination occurs when microorganisms are transferred from one body area to another, which can cause infection in a previously non-infected area. Changing gloves when caring for wounds on different parts of the body can prevent auto contamination.

A is incorrect because although handwashing can prevent infection, it will not prevent auto contamination.

C is incorrect because using a disposable blood pressure cuff will not prevent auto contamination.

D is incorrect because the closed method of burn wound management will not prevent auto contamination.

34. The nurse has provided burn prevention education to a group at the community center. Which of the following statements by the community members indicates the nurse needs to provide more education?

    A. "My chimney gets swept every other year by a professional."
    B. "When the temperature reaches zero, I use a space heater."

C. "My home hot water heater is set to 120 degrees."

D. "It's ok for me to smoke when I wake up throughout the night."

Rationale:

Correct answer: D

House fires are common and can lead to serious injury and death. Smoking at night is a serious danger and the nurse should ask the person more about this habit, as falling asleep with a lit cigarette in the bed poses a major risk. Smokers should be taught to smoke outside and use wide, sturdy ashtrays. Other common causes of house fires include unattended candles and overloaded electrical sockets.

A is incorrect because although it is recommended to have chimneys swept annually, this not as dangerous as smoking in bed.

B is incorrect because space heaters should be used with caution, but they are not as dangerous as smoking in bed.

C is incorrect because water heaters should be set below 140 degrees to decrease risk for house fire. It is also important to teach about regularly cleaning the lint trap in the dryer and keeping the laundry area free from combustible material and flammable chemicals.

35. The nurse is assessing patients in the emergency room. Which of the following patients requires immediate intervention by the nurse?

   A. Patient who has copious drainage from an incision
   B. Patient whose pulse oximetry is 92% on 2L of oxygen
   C. Patient who rates incisional pain as a 6 out of 10
   D. Patient whose trachea is deviated

Rationale:

Correct answer: D

A deviated trachea indicates a possible tension pneumothorax. This is a medical emergency that requires immediate intervention to prevent cardiac and respiratory arrest. Tension pneumothorax occurs when air escapes into the pleural space, placing pressure on the lungs and forcing the affected lung to the opposite side, which deviates the trachea and compromises airway and cardiac function.

A is incorrect because, although copious drainage is not expected and needs to be investigated by the nurse, this is circulatory or infection-related and does not take priority over breathing.

B is incorrect because oxygen saturation of 92% is not life threatening and doesn't pose as much of a threat as a deviated trachea.

C is incorrect because pain 6 out of 10 does not take priority over other patients with greater physical concerns.

36. The nurse is caring for a patient recovering from anterior cervical discectomy and fusion. When the assessment is performed, which of the following findings should be reported to the healthcare provider immediately?

    A. Stridor heard on auscultation
    B. Difficulty swallowing
    C. Inability to shrug shoulders
    D. Weak pedal pulses

Rationale:

Correct answer: A

Stridor indicates narrowing of the trachea due to postoperative swelling. This can cause a partial airway obstruction and requires immediate notification of the healthcare provider.

B is incorrect because trouble swallowing may be due to postoperative swelling, but the airway is priority. If the patient has trouble swallowing, the nurse should keep the patient NPO and reassess to see if swallowing ability improves as anesthesia wears off.

C is incorrect because inability to shrug shoulders is a sign that cervical nerves may have been damaged, but this is not more concerning than stridor.

D is incorrect because weak pedal pulses are not a complication of the surgery. This may indicate dehydration or circulatory compromise, but airway takes priority.

37. A patient is admitted to the pre-operative area for total joint replacement. Which action is most important for perioperative staff for preventing surgical wound infection?

    A. Administer a preoperative antibiotic intravenously
    B. Administer a preoperative antibiotic PO
    C. Instruct the patient to shower the night before
    D. Monitor the patient's temperature postoperatively

Rationale:

Correct answer: A

Antibiotics are given by IV prophylactically before surgery within an hour of the first incision to prevent surgical site infection postoperatively.

B is incorrect because PO meds should not be administered preoperatively because the patient should be NPO.

C is incorrect because prophylactic antibiotics are more important for infection prevention than showering the night before. A shower will not prevent infection unless special antimicrobial soap is used.

D is incorrect because it will identify when an infection is occurring, not prevent it.

38. A patient who had hip replacement surgery is under the care of a nurse. What is the most important action by the nurse to prevent wound infection?

    A. Assess the patient's white blood cell count
    B. Culture any drainage from the wound
    C. Monitor the patient's temperature every four hours
    D. Use aseptic technique for dressing changes

Rationale:

Correct answer: D

The nurse has primary responsibility for preventing surgical site infection. Using aseptic technique for changing the dressing can prevent infection.

A is incorrect because monitoring white blood cell count will not prevent surgical wound infection. Elevated WBC is a sign of infection, but not a prevention measure.

B is incorrect because culturing drainage is necessary to identify causative organism but will not prevent surgical wound infection.

C is incorrect because elevated temperature may indicate infection is occurring, not prevent it.

39. A patient who underwent an uncemented hip replacement procedure is getting out of bed and into the chair for the first time since the surgery. What is the most important action by the nurse?

    A. Request assistance from the UAP to transfer the patient
    B. Provide socks so the patient can slide easier
    C. Tell the patient that partial weight-bearing is allowed on the affected leg
    D. Use a footstool to elevate the patient's leg while sitting in the chair

Rationale:

Correct answer: A

A patient who has an uncemented hip will be unable to place any weight on the affected side. In order to prevent injury and falls, the nurse should make sure to have enough help to safely transfer the patient to the chair.

B is incorrect because socks can lead to a fall.

C is incorrect because the patient should not bear any weight on the affected leg.

D is incorrect because a 90-degree angle of the hip joint is contraindicated after hip replacement surgery.

40. A patient with suspected bacterial meningitis is interviewed by the emergency room nurse. Which of the following questions should the nurse ask for a focused health history?

    A. "Do you live in a crowded residence?"
    B. "When was your last tetanus vaccination?"
    C. "Have you experienced any viral infections recently?"
    D. "Have you traveled outside of the country in the last month?"

Rationale:

Correct answer: A

Bacterial meningitis usually occurs in outbreaks. It is often found in high-density population areas such as college dorms, prisons, and military barracks.

B is incorrect because a tetanus vaccination does not cause increased risk for meningitis nor prevent meningitis.

C is incorrect because viral infections do not lead to bacterial meningitis, but viral meningitis.

D is incorrect because the question does not provide enough information unless asking about specific countries where the disease is common. Most U.S. cases of meningitis are not caused by foreign travel. (The highest incidence of the disease globally is in the "Meningitis-belt" of Sub-Saharan Africa: Ethiopia, Southern Sudan, Chad, Niger, Nigeria, Burkina Faso, Mali, and Guinea.)

41. A patient has 24-hour electrocardiography with a Holter monitor placed for frequent fainting spells. In order to prevent electrical interference, the nurse instructs the patient to avoid which of the following?

    A. Use of a microwave oven
    B. Use of an electric razor
    C. Driving under power lines
    D. Use of headphones

Rationale:

Correct answer: B

A Holter monitor is worn by a patient for 24 hours to record cardiac activity and identify what causes fainting spells, palpitations, or chest pain. The patient keeps a diary of activities whenever they notice something unusual, which later can be interpreted by the ECG from the Holter monitor readings to identify the problem.

Some household electrical devices including electric razors, electric blankets, and electric toothbrushes can interfere with data recorded by a Holter monitor. It is important to teach the patient not to swim or bathe when wearing the Holter monitor, and to keep the device and its wires dry at all times.

A is incorrect because a microwave oven will not interfere with a Holter monitor. Patients with pacemakers are cautioned about standing in close proximity to a microwave when in use because the electromagnetic energy from the microwave can leak and affect the function of the pacemaker.

C is incorrect because power lines do not interfere with a Holter monitor.

D is incorrect because use of headphones is not contraindicated. A cell phone or MP3 player may interfere with a Holter monitor, so patients should be encouraged to keep these devices at least six inches away from their chest.

42. The day shift nurse is charting on a patient and finds the night shift nurse did not complete documentation of patient care completed on the shift. What is the best action by the nurse to fix the documentation issue?

    A. Forgive the night shift nurse due to fatigue
    B. Leave space for the night shift nurse to continue documentation tonight
    C. Call the nurse and have the note dictated over the phone
    D. Cross out the entry and note the night nurse will document separately

Rationale:

Correct answer: C

Notes can be dictated by nurses just as verbal orders from other healthcare providers can be taken. The day shift nurse should call the night shift nurse and document the note.

A is incorrect because the documentation needs to be completed.

B is incorrect because leaving space allows for entry of incorrect information.

D is incorrect because crossing out an entry with a line indicates an error.

43. The school nurse is observing children at recess on the playground. Which of the following observations would most concern the nurse?

    A. A 5-year-old tugging at their ear, crying and squeezing a stuffed animal

    B. Children pulling at each other on a swing

    C. A 4-year-old bent over with mouth wide open, tongue stuck out and drooling

    D. Children fighting over a ball

Rationale:

Correct answer: C

The child bent over with mouth wide open and tongue stuck out may have epiglottitis or inflammation of the epiglottis which threatens the child's airway. This is the most concerning observation by the nurse and requires immediate intervention.

A is incorrect because the symptoms are consistent with ear infection or earache, which does not require immediate intervention.

B is incorrect because while pulling at each other on a swing is a risk for injury, it does not require immediate intervention.

D is incorrect because fighting over a ball is expected behavior among children and does not require immediate intervention.

44. At shift report, the night shift nurse tells the day shift nurse a new patient is on seizure precautions. Which of the following interventions by the day shift nurse is appropriate?

    A. Serve meals on paper plates with plastic dinnerware

    B. Apply soft limb restraints to the patient's arms

    C. Keep the bed in the lowest position

    D. Transfer the patient to a room at the end of the hall so the patient can rest

Rationale:

Correct answer: C

When a patient is on seizure precautions, the bed should be in the lowest position. This will decrease the risk of injury should the patient experience a seizure and fall out of bed. Side rails should be up and padded.

A is incorrect because paper and plastic dinnerware are not necessary for the patient on seizure precautions.

B is incorrect because soft limb restraints are inappropriate for a patient on seizure precautions and can increase risk for injury.

D is incorrect because the patient should be visualized frequently while on seizure precautions and thus, should be close to the nurse's station.

45. The nurse is caring for a patient who has had a myelogram. Which of the following assessments is most important to be performed by the nurse for patient safety?

    A. Make sure the patient lies flat after the procedure for two hours
    B. Check bilateral popliteal pulses
    C. Ensure the patient signed the consent form
    D. Perform a neurological assessment

Rationale:

Correct answer: D

Contrast dye is injected into the spine during a myelogram in order to visualize the spinal cord. A needle is placed into the spinal cord for this, so it is imperative to perform a neurological assessment in order to identify any impaired or altered sensation or function.

A is incorrect because a patient should not lie completely flat after a myelogram because it could cause seizures. A lumbar puncture requires the patient to lie flat for six hours after the procedure.

B is incorrect because popliteal pulses do not indicate neurological function. A myelogram does not impair circulation.

C is incorrect because the consent should be signed before the procedure.

46. A patient is admitted to the emergency room with suspected appendicitis. Which of the following actions by the unlicensed assistive personnel (UAP) requires intervention by the nurse?

    A. The UAP maintains the patient's NPO status
    B. The UAP gives the patient a heat pack
    C. The UAP encourages the patient to lie in a comfortable position
    D. The UAP tells the patient to stay in bed

Rationale:

Correct answer: B

Heating pads, enemas, and laxatives are contraindicated for a patient with appendicitis.

A is incorrect because the patient with suspected appendicitis should be maintained NPO. IV fluids are given to prevent dehydration.

C is incorrect because the patient should lie in whichever position is most comfortable. Drawing the knees toward the chest may be very painful.

D is incorrect because the patient should stay in bed to prevent a fall due to the severity of pain associated with appendicitis.

47. A patient with moderate stage Alzheimer's disease is visited by the home health nurse. The patient is slightly confused and lives with their son- and daughter-in-law. Which of the following observations made by the nurse is most concerning?

    A. The door has a deadbolt near the doorknob
    B. Extension cords are on the floor, secured behind furniture
    C. Rugs are secured to the floor
    D. Stovetops must be activated with a hidden switch

Rationale:

Correct answer: A

Home safety is critical for a patient with Alzheimer's or another dementia. In a home with an Alzheimer's patient, doors leading to the exterior of the house should have locks placed in atypical locations such as at the top of the door. This will prevent the confused patient from exiting the house at night and wandering outside unattended. Patients can get lost on their own streets or even in their own homes.

B is incorrect because the extension cords do not pose a safety hazard if they are secured behind furniture. Walkways should also remain well lit and floors should be clutter-free.

C is incorrect because the rugs do not pose a safety hazard if they are safely secured. Alzheimer's patients may have a poor sense of balance and may depend on a walker to move about the home.

D is incorrect because stovetops need a hidden switch for activation to prevent injury in the event that the confused patient tries to turn on the appliance. Alzheimer's can affect a patient's sense of judgment and ability to use household equipment.

48. The nurse and an unlicensed assistive personnel (UAP) are caring for a patient with left-sided paralysis. Which of the following actions by the UAP requires intervention by the nurse?

    A. The UAP places their hand in the patient's left axilla when helping the nurse move the patient up in the bed

B. The UAP places the gait belt around the patient's waist before getting them up for ambulation

C. The UAP encourages the patient to perform activities of daily living (ADLs) independently

D. The UAP places the patient on her back in bed with head turned and HOB elevated 45 degrees

Rationale:

Correct answer: A

The nurse should intervene when the UAP attempts to use the axilla for repositioning the patient in bed as this could cause shoulder dislocation. A lift sheet should always be used when repositioning a hemiparetic patient in bed. This provides for both patient and healthcare worker safety.

B is incorrect because it is an appropriate action. The purpose of the gait belt is to provide increased security for the patient and staff and prevent injury during gait training and transferring of the patient. Gait belts are contraindicated in patients with recent rib fracture, recent surgery in the area of the belt, a gastrostomy tube, hiatal hernia, a colostomy, or severe heart or respiratory disease.

C is incorrect because the nursing team should encourage patients to stay as independent as possible. Hemiparesis does not incapacitate the patient. Even if the dominant side is affected, the patient should be encouraged to perform ADLs using the non-dominant hand.

D is incorrect because it is an appropriate action. Elevating the HOB facilitates easy breathing and turning the head to the side decreases the risk of aspiration if the patient has a productive cough.

49. The nurse on the medical-surgical unit is caring for a patient who has Meniere's disease. For patient safety, the nurse recognizes the most important intervention for this patient is:

   A. Encourage the patient to perform hand hygiene after going to the bathroom and before eating

   B. Allow the patient to make alternative meal choices

   C. Keep the side rails on the bed raised

   D. Assist the patient with ambulation

Rationale:

Correct answer: D

Meniere's disease is an inner ear disorder that causes vertigo and hearing loss. Vertigo can occur quite rapidly so the patient should be assisted with ambulation to prevent a fall.

A is incorrect because handwashing is an appropriate intervention but not related to safety.

B is incorrect because alternative meal choices are appropriate but not related to safety. All patients should be given the option to choose their food options within the prescribed diet. This fosters a sense of independence and control over their hospital stay.

C is incorrect because raised side rails are a form of restraint and inappropriate for the Meniere's patient. The patient should be instructed to call for help when getting in and out of bed to prevent falling.

50. The night shift nurse is caring for an older patient in the intensive care unit (ICU) who had heart surgery two days ago and is now disoriented and trying to climb out of the bed. What is the most important intervention for this patient to prevent injury?

    A. Apply soft wrist restraints to keep the patient in bed
    B. Administer a sleep aid to help the patient sleep
    C. Move the patient to a room close to the nurse's station
    D. Notify the healthcare provider of an order for an antipsychotic medication

Rationale:

Correct answer: C

Anesthesia often causes disorientation after surgery, especially in older patients, as it takes longer for the body to process and excrete the byproducts of the medication. This, coupled with lack of sleep due to constant stimulation and lights in the ICU, can contribute to delirium and increases patient safety concerns. The patient should be moved to a room close to the nurse's station so they can be visualized at all times.

A is incorrect because wrist restraints could agitate the patient further and cause injury. The nurse should only use restraints if a less-restrictive option is unavailable.

B is incorrect because sleep aids often worsen disorientation.

D is incorrect because an antipsychotic medication may not relieve the disorientation and worsen the quality of sleep. The nurse should always attempt non-pharmacologic measures first.

51. The nurse is caring for a confused patient who is continually pulling at their IV tubing. The patient pulls out a peripheral IV, and the nurse places a new IV. In order to maintain patient safety, which type of restraint should the nurse use?

    A. Mitts placed on both of the patient's hands
    B. Bilateral soft wrist restraints
    C. Soft wrist and ankle restraints

D. Mitt placed on the hand opposite the extremity with the IV

Rationale:

Correct answer: D

Mitts are special padded gloves with mesh on the back that are used to prevent undesired removal of tubes or dressings. The least restrictive measure should be used to achieve the desired outcome for the patient. One or two mitts can be used, but in this case, only one is needed. A mitt restraint allows the patient to move the extremity but prevents the patient from using their fingers to pull at the IV. This is the least restrictive and most appropriate restraint for patient safety.

A is incorrect because mitts on both hands are not needed and may agitate the patient.

B is incorrect because soft wrist restraints restrict mobility of the upper extremities and are more restrictive than mitts. This patient only needs the hand opposite the IV to be restrained.

C is incorrect because 4-point restraints are not the least amount of restraint and are inappropriate for this patient.

52. A patient has a CT scan with contrast ordered for this afternoon. The nurse knows the most important action to be performed for patient safety is:

    A. Raise the side rails of the bed
    B. Review the patient's allergies
    C. Ensure the consent is signed
    D. Encourage PO fluids once the patient returns from the CT scan

Rationale:

Correct answer: B

Contrast dye utilized in CT contains iodine. The nurse must review the patient's allergies to check for sensitivity to iodine or shellfish to prevent an allergic reaction.

A is incorrect because raising side rails is restrictive and is not the most important action. Side rails that are raised can be used to prevent a patient falling from the bed but should only be used when necessary. This is not standard practice for a patient scheduled for a CT.

C is incorrect because although it is important to make sure the consent is signed, it is not the most important action and does not ensure patient safety.

D is incorrect because, although it is important to encourage fluids to increase renal clearance of the contrast medium, it is not the most important action.

53. The nurse cares for a 75-year-old male patient recovering from prostatectomy for benign prostatic hypertrophy. Before surgery, the patient was alert and oriented, and several hours after surgery he is confused and agitated and trying to climb out of bed. What is the most appropriate action the nurse should implement to calm the patient?

    A. Limit visits by the family
    B. Encourage the family to call on the phone
    C. Move the patient to a well-lit and active area
    D. Speak with a soothing tone of voice and play quiet music

Rationale:

Correct answer: D

A patient who is confused and agitated can be calmed with a soothing, quiet tone of voice and quiet music. Frequent rounds by the nurse should be performed to reorient the patient and prevent injury.

A is incorrect because family can help reorient the patient and keep him calm. Visitors should not be discouraged unless the patient is in isolation or displaying threatening behavior that poses a risk to others.

B is incorrect because a confused patient often becomes more confused by taking a phone call. Direct face-to-face interaction is best for reorienting the patient. Phone calls will likely not prevent the patient from climbing out of bed.

C is incorrect because the patient who is confused needs a calm, quiet environment. Overstimulation can worsen agitation.

54. The home health nurse is visiting an elderly patient and assessing risk for falls. The most important factor the nurse should consider is:

    A. Lighting in the home
    B. Whether or not the patient is getting regular exercise
    C. The patient's resting heart rate
    D. Salt intake

Rationale:

Correct answer: A

The most important factor to consider in a home assessment is lighting. To prevent falls, lighting should be appropriate including night lights if the patient gets up at night. Other factors to consider include power cords (should be tucked behind furniture), rugs (should be eliminated from the home or secured to the floor), spills, and bathroom handrails. The home should be clutter-free to allow for easy mobility.

B is incorrect because exercise can be beneficial to prevent falls, but not the most important factor.

C is incorrect because resting heart rate is not related to preventing a fall.

D is incorrect because salt intake is not directly related to preventing a fall. Hyponatremia may cause nausea and muscle cramps. Hypernatremia may cause weakness and disorientation, which could contribute to risk for falls, but assessing lighting in the home is more important.

55. A 79-year-old patient with macular degeneration is admitted to the preoperative area prior to surgery. Preoperative goals for the patient assigned by the nurse should include:

    A. Independent ambulation
    B. Reading educational materials
    C. Safe maneuvering around the hospital room
    D. Using a bedside commode

Rationale:

Correct answer: C

Macular degeneration is characterized by blurry vision or loss of vision in the center of the visual field due to deterioration of the retina. Patients with macular degeneration may have difficulty recognizing faces, driving, reading, or performing other activities of daily living. It is important for the nurse to orient the patient to the room so that they can maneuver around the room safely both before and after surgery.

A is incorrect because independent ambulation post-operatively is inappropriate for this patient and could result in an injury or fall. The patient will need assistance with ambulation as the eyes heal after surgery.

B is incorrect because patients with macular degeneration may have difficulty reading educational materials. The best way to teach the patient about pre-operative care and post-operative expectations is for the nurse to talk one-on-one with the patient and provide direct teaching, allowing for questions.

D is incorrect because it is an unnecessary restriction and inappropriate for this patient. The patient should be able to ambulate to the bathroom with assistance after surgery and void in the toilet.

56. A 3-year-old is admitted to the pediatric intensive care unit (PICU) with febrile seizures. When preparing the patient's room, which action by the nurse is most important?

A. Drawing lab work and monitor white blood cell count

B. Placing a urine specimen cup in the bathroom

C. Preparing ice packs

D. Placing padding on the side rails

Rationale:

Correct answer: D

A patient admitted with febrile seizures requires the nurse to implement safety precautions to prevent injury. The nurse should place padding on the side rails, so if the child has a seizure in the bed, injury from the hard side rails is prevented. Other important components of seizure precautions include placing the bed in the lowest position and providing a quiet environment.

A is incorrect because blood testing is not the most important and is not a component of room preparation.

B is incorrect because a urine specimen is not necessarily related to seizure precautions.

C is incorrect because rapid cooling measures such as tepid sponging, fanning, and ice packs are no longer recommended for children. Antipyretics are usually administered rectally for febrile seizures. Cool PO fluids, if tolerated, can also be used to cool the child, and prevent dehydration.

57. A nursing student is preparing to administer an intramuscular (IM) injection of morphine to a patient complaining of pain. Which of the following actions by the student requires intervention by the nurse?

A. Recapping the needle using both hands

B. Using aseptic technique to draw up the medication

C. Wearing gloves to find the appropriate injection site

D. Using the Z-track method for injection

Rationale:

Correct answer: A

Needles should never be recapped whether they have been used to draw up medications or to administer an injection. When performing an IM injection, the medication is drawn up with one needle, which is then discarded in the sharps container to be replaced with the needle for the IM injection. Once the injection is given, the needle and syringe are discarded in the sharps container. Recapping a needle puts the student at risk for a needlestick injury.

B is incorrect because using aseptic technique to draw up medications is appropriate.

C is incorrect because, although wearing gloves to locate an injection site is not required, this does not pose a threat to the patient or the student.

D is incorrect because the Z-track method is appropriate for IM injections to prevent drainage of medication through subcutaneous tissue once the needle is withdrawn, and also decreases likelihood of causing a skin lesion at the injection site. The tissue should not be massaged after a Z-track injection.

58. A 44-year-old patient who is blind and deaf is admitted to the medical-surgical unit. The primary responsibility of the charge nurse is which of the following?

   A. Communicate the patient's deficits to all other healthcare workers on the unit
   B. Communicate safety concerns to the nursing supervisor
   C. Keep the patient updated about changes in the environment
   D. Ensure a safe and secure patient environment

Rationale:

Correct answer: D

When providing care for a patient who is blind and deaf, safety is the primary concern. The nurse must find out the best way to communicate with the patient and put safety measures in place to prevent patient injury and falls.

A is incorrect because the healthcare workers on the unit only need to be aware of the patient's deficits if they are providing care to that patient. Patient confidentiality must be maintained by sharing personal and medical information only with those directly involved in care of the patient.

B is incorrect because communicating safety concerns to the nursing supervisor does not promote a safe environment. The charge nurse should implement safety measures to eliminate safety concerns.

C is incorrect because the environment should not change. The patient must be oriented to the room upon arrival. And all furniture and equipment should remain in place in order for the patient to remain oriented.

59. The nurse is caring for four patients on the medical unit. Which of the following patients does the nurse need to place on airborne precautions?

   A. Patient with AIDS and cytomegalovirus
   B. Patient with suspected viral pneumonia
   C. Patient with advanced lung cancer
   D. Patient who had a positive PPD and abnormal chest X-ray

Rationale:

Correct answer: D

The purified protein derivative (PPD) is administered as a subcutaneous injection to test for a reaction to tuberculin. A patient who has a positive PPD and an abnormal chest X-ray is suspected of having tuberculosis (TB) and would need to be placed in a negative airflow room on airborne precautions.

A is incorrect because AIDS and cytomegalovirus require standard precautions.

B is incorrect because viral pneumonia requires droplet precautions.

C is incorrect because advanced lung cancer requires standard precautions.

60. A 28-year-old patient is being discharged from the hospital after a new diagnosis of acquired immune deficiency syndrome (AIDS). The nurse has taught the patient about prevention of transmission of AIDS. Which patient statement indicates the teaching was understood?

   A. "I will not touch my 5-year-old niece."
   B. "I can no longer play soccer."
   C. "I must use protection for sexual intercourse."
   D. "I will drop my classes at the university."

Rationale:

Correct answer: C

AIDS is spread through direct contact with blood and body fluids, including through sexual intercourse. The patient must use a barrier protection during sexual intercourse to prevent spreading AIDS to their sexual partner. The nurse should also educate the patient about avoiding IV drug use (sharing needles), consuming a diet high in protein and calories, and not sharing toothbrushes or razors. The patient must be encouraged to seek support from others who live with AIDS as they learn to cope with this long-term illness.

A is incorrect because casual contact does not risk transmission of HIV. The niece is only at increased risk for infection with HIV if she is immunocompromised.

B is incorrect because contact sports are only contraindicated if there are significant chances for bleeding and contact with other players. Soccer is high-impact but not a high-contact sport. The patient with AIDS should be encouraged to remain active and social while adjusting to life with this new diagnosis. Preventing social isolation is an important goal.

D is incorrect because the patient can continue attending classes unless they feel ill.

61. Before finishing the night shift on the medical-surgical unit, which of the following actions is most important for the nurse to complete?

    A. Emptying the trash and linen receptacles in the patients' rooms
    B. Restocking supplies at the bedside
    C. Changing bed linens
    D. Documenting care provided

Rationale:

Correct answer: D

As the shift is coming to an end, the nurse must document all the care provided during that shift. This is the only legal way to claim interventions were performed. Documentation of nursing care cannot be delegated. Documentation should be thorough, factual, descriptive, and objective.

A is incorrect because this is a task that can be delegated and it not more important than documentation.

B is incorrect because documentation is the priority. Restocking supplies can be done by assistive personnel.

C is incorrect because bed linens do not need to be changed at the end of a shift. Linens should be changed at the time the patient is bathed or when otherwise soiled. This is also a task that can be delegated to support staff such as an LPN/LVN or a UAP.

62. The nurse is teaching the parents of a 9-year-old. Which of the following topics is highest priority?

    A. Dispel fears with use of a nightlight
    B. Body integrity fears are normal
    C. Encourage independence of the child
    D. Accident prevention

Rationale:

Correct answer: D

Accidents are a major cause of injury and death to school-age children. Accident prevention should be highest priority when teaching these parents. The nurse should include the following instructions for accident prevention with school-age children: don't smoke near children, be sure the home is free from lead-based paint, wear a helmet when riding a bike, rollerblading, or skateboarding, keep the poison control hotline number visible near the phone, teach children to obey traffic signals when walking or riding a bike, keep water heater at no more than 120°F, and teach swimming safety.

A is incorrect because accident prevention is more important. School-age children may fear the dark, death, injury, and being alone. When hospitalized, pre-school and school-aged children should be allowed to play with medical equipment (when appropriate and within limits) and ask questions so they understand the care being provided.

B is incorrect because school-age children are generally not concerned about body integrity. Alteration in body image is a common fear of adolescents, especially when having surgery.

C is incorrect accident prevention is a greater priority. School-age children may experience fear of loss of control when hospitalized, so the nurse should explain care in simple terms and allow the child to make choices when possible.

63. The nurse is teaching a 4-year-old child's parents about accidental poisoning in the home. Which of the following should the nurse instruct the parents to perform first if their child ingests poison?

    A. Give the child syrup of ipecac

    B. Call poison control

    C. Administer an emetic and save the vomit

    D. Call for an ambulance

Rationale:

Correct answer: B

Poison control should be called first and the parent should be prepared to give information about the substance (name amount, time, and route) and the child's age, weight. Instructions will be given for how to treat the child at home, and whether to take the child to an emergency facility.

A is incorrect because syrup of ipecac is no longer indicated for poison treatment at home, and all ipecac solutions in homes should be discarded.

C is incorrect because an emetic should not be administered unless directed by Poison Control. If the child does vomit, the vomit (and/or urine, stool) should be saved in the event it needs to be analyzed to determine what substance was ingested.

D is incorrect because, although the ambulance may need to be called, it is not the first action the parents should perform.

(Note: Other important components when teaching about poisoning are to keep all poisonous substances and medications locked away in an out-of-reach area from children, closely supervise young children, leave medicines and cleaning supplies in original containers, and keep the poison control hotline number near phone.)

64. The charge nurse of the medical-surgical unit is reviewing infection control procedures. While observing the healthcare workers, which of the following observations indicates a need for staff education?

    A. The LPN changes gloves multiple times when giving a patient a bath
    B. A patient admitted with active TB does not have a mask placed when leaving the room for testing
    C. The nurse dons a mask, gown, and gloves before entering a strict isolation room
    D. The unlicensed assistive personnel (UAP) feeds a patient without wearing gloves

Rationale:

Correct answer: B

The patient with active TB must wear a mask when leaving the negative airflow room for testing. This will prevent the spread of TB, as it is airborne. The nurse caring for this patient requires more education regarding infection control.

A is incorrect because this is an appropriate action. Gloves may need to be changed several times during a bath to prevent contaminating clean areas of the patient's body after coming into contact with body fluids.

C is incorrect because when entering a strict isolation room, the nurse should don a mask, gown, and gloves. This is an appropriate action.

D is incorrect because feeding a patient does not require use of gloves unless the patient is on specific precautions or the patient has open wounds near the mouth, so this is an appropriate action.

65. The nurse is caring for a patient admitted with methicillin resistant staphylococcus aureus (MRSA) pneumonia. The nurse knows the most appropriate isolation is which of the following?

    A. Standard precautions
    B. Respiratory isolation
    C. Contact isolation
    D. Reverse isolation

Rationale:

Correct answer: C

Whenever determining the most appropriate isolation to utilize for a patient with infection, the mode of transmission is considered. MRSA is transmitted by dirty hands, and as this patient has pneumonia, there is a need for precautions with sputum. The nurse should place the patient in a private room and don gloves, mask, gown, and protective eyewear as appropriate. Strict handwashing technique is also required.

Contact precautions are also required for herpes simplex, herpes zoster, *Clostridium difficile*, respiratory syncytial virus (RSV), scabies, pediculosis, rotavirus, and hepatitis A. Clean, non-sterile gloves must be worn for any activity that requires contact with the patient or the patient's linens or belongings. Dedicated equipment (*e.g.,* stethoscope) should be used for infected patients or disinfected after each use. Gown should be worn when entering a room if clothing may come into contact with the infected patient or environmental surfaces (bedrails, bedside table, commode, lavatory surfaces in patient's bathroom, doorknobs, telephone, call light) in the patient's room.

A is incorrect because standard precautions are insufficient for caring for the patient with MRSA pneumonia. Standard precautions must be used in addition to contact precautions when caring for a patient with a drug-resistant organism.

B is incorrect because respiratory isolation is not needed for the patient with MRSA pneumonia.

D is incorrect because reverse isolation is not needed for the patient with MRSA pneumonia. Reverse isolation is used to prevent an immunocompromised patient from becoming infected with a pathogen or disease-causing agent.

66. The nurse is evaluating the LPN/LVN's knowledge regarding prevention of transmission of human immunodeficiency virus (HIV). Which of the following behaviors by the LPN/LVN demonstrates correct understanding of standard precautions?

   A. The LPN/LVN recaps the needle after drawing blood
   B. The LPN/LVN wears gloves to feed an elderly patient
   C. The LPN/LVN dons a mask and protective eyewear before assisting with tracheostomy suctioning
   D. The LPN/LVN refuses to assist in the care of a patient with acquired immunodeficiency syndrome (AIDS)

Rationale:

Correct answer: C

Suctioning a tracheostomy requires donning of a mask and protective eyewear for droplet production during coughing. The sputum may contain blood, so donning protective eyewear and a mask is safe practice for preventing transmission of HIV. Standard precautions are guidelines recommended by the Centers for Disease Control and Prevention to reduce the risk of transmission of blood-borne and other pathogens in healthcare settings. Standard precautions apply to blood and all body secretions and excretions (except sweat), mucous membranes, and non-intact skin.

A is incorrect because needles should never be recapped regardless of the patient's diagnosis. Recapping needles leads to needle-stick injury.

B is incorrect because gloves are not required for feeding a patient unless the patient is on specific precautions or the patient has open wounds near the mouth.

D is incorrect because as long as standard precautions are followed, the risk of transmission of HIV is extremely low.

67. The nurse is teaching a patient about changing a sterile dressing on their leg. Which of the following patient statements indicates correct understanding regarding maintaining asepsis?

    A. "If I drop the bandages on the floor, they can still be used if not soiled."
    B. "If I drop the bandages on the floor, they can be rinsed with sterile normal saline."
    C. "If I don't think any of the dressing material is sterile, I won't use it."
    D. "I should put on the sterile gloves first, then open the bottle of saline for soaking the bandages."

Rationale:

Correct answer: C

If the sterility of any dressing material or instrument is questionable, it should not be used. This will prevent contamination of the wound.

A is incorrect because dressing materials dropped on the floor are no longer sterile and shouldn't be used.

B is incorrect because rinsing in sterile saline will not re-sterilize the dressing material. If dropped on the floor, items should be discarded.

D is incorrect because the bandages should be soaked in sterile saline or sterile water before putting on sterile gloves.

68. A patient returns to the emergency room complaining of severe pain and numb toes after a long leg cast was placed the previous day. The healthcare provider removes the cast; however, the patient still complains of severe pain. Which of the following does the nurse suspect?

    A. Pressure ulcer
    B. Fat embolism
    C. Infection

D. Compartment syndrome

Rationale:

Correction answer: D

Compartment syndrome is the result of excessive pressure built up in an enclosed muscle space, usually due to bleeding or swelling after injury. This excessive pressure impacts blood flow into and out of the affected tissue, in this case, the leg, and requires fasciotomy surgery to release the pressure and prevent permanent injury. Compartment syndrome is a neuromuscular medical emergency and can lead to loss of limb if not treated within 4-6 hours. Signs of compartment syndrome include severe pain that is unrelieved despite pain medication, lack of pulse, pallor, numbness, and tingling.

A is incorrect because the cast has not been in place long enough to cause a pressure ulcer and the symptoms (numb toes and severe pain) do not correlate with a pressure ulcer.

B is incorrect because severe pain and numbness are not signs of a fat embolism. A patient with a long bone fracture *is*, however, at risk for a fat embolism which can escape from the yellow marrow cavity within the bone and travel to another part of the body, such as the lungs (causing a pulmonary embolism) or the brain (causing stroke symptoms.)

C is incorrect because severe pain and numb toes are not indicative of infection. Infection presents with redness, oozing from the wound, elevated temperature, and elevated serum WBCs.

69. A child on the orthopedic unit calls the nurse and complains about the cast placed on their leg earlier today. Which of the following statements by the child require immediate intervention by the nurse?

    A. "Can I get something to scratch inside the cast?"
    B. "My leg is itchy."
    C. "This cast edge hurts."
    D. "My leg feels weird."

Rationale:

Correct answer: D

Weird is a vague term requiring the nurse to gather more assessment data. Although it may be a normal description of how the leg feels, this child may be experiencing paresthesia, or impaired sensation, which can occur as a result of the cast being too tight on the leg. The cast may need to be removed and replaced to prevent further injury to the leg.

A is incorrect because the potential paresthesia is of greater concern. The nurse should teach the patient that nothing should be stuck inside the cast to relieve itching because skin breakdown can occur or an item can become lodged in the cast. Patients at home will often use an item such as a pen, coat hanger, or tongue depressor to reach into the cast and relieve itching. If the skin is pierced, this can lead to infection, which might go unnoticed because the skin is concealed by the cast.

B is incorrect because itching does not require immediate intervention. Itching is often caused by excess moisture within the cast. The patient can be educated about safe ways to relieve itching: a small amount of talcum powder may be able to be applied under the cast, a hairdryer set on the coolest setting can help dry the moisture within the cast, or antihistamines can be taken orally to relieve the itching.

C is incorrect because a rough-cast edge does not require immediate intervention. The padding under the outer surface of the cast should extend beyond the cast to prevent discomfort.

70. A 64-year-old patient is admitted to the emergency department for urinary retention. When the nurse performs the bladder scan, the result is 1800 mL. The nurse knows that when straight catheterizing the patient, the most important intervention during the procedure is:

    A. Clamping the drainage tube after 500 mL intervals and wait five minutes
    B. Educate the patient about urinary retention
    C. Teach the patient sterile self-catheterization technique
    D. Have the patient attempt to void after draining 500 mL with the catheter

Rationale:

Correct answer: A

In order to prevent bladder spasms, the nurse should clamp the drainage tube after 500 mL intervals and wait several minutes before continuing to drain the bladder.

B is incorrect because teaching is important but not the most important intervention.

C is incorrect because the patient may not need to self-catheterize, and this intervention increases the risk for infection.

D is incorrect because the patient cannot void with the catheter in place and removing the catheter can cause swelling of the urethra, compounding urinary retention.

71. The nurse in the pediatric emergency room is triaging patients. Which of the following manifestations in a 3-month-old Hispanic infant concerns the nurse the most?

A. Irregular-shaped pale pink patches at the back of the neck

B. A bluish-purple bruised area on the buttock

C. Slightly bulging anterior fontanel when the child is crying

D. Raised, demarcated, dark red cluster of capillaries on left eyelid

Rationale:

Correct answer: D

This describes a hemangioma, which often is benign. However, hemangiomas near the eyes, nose, lips, and ears can irreversibly damage underlying cartilage. A hemangioma near the eye can also impair vision and disturb normal eye development leading to deprivation amblyopia.

A is incorrect because the pink patches describe telangiectatic nevi (also known as "stork bites") which are clusters of capillaries that blanch with finger pressure. They are commonly found on the eyelids, nose, or nape of the neck, and they usually fade during infancy. No intervention is required.

B is incorrect because the bluish-purple area describes a Mongolian spot (bluish or dark gray non-elevated skin pigmentation on lower back or buttocks), most commonly seen in Hispanic, African American, and Asian babies.

C is incorrect because this is expected. If the fontanel bulges while the baby is at rest, or if the bulging is constant, this can indicate increased intracranial pressure. The anterior fontanel usually closes completely by 18 months of age.

72. The nurse has administered pain medication to a patient who sustained a crush injury to the arm. One hour after the medication was administered, the patient continues to complain of severe pain. Which action by the nurse is most appropriate?

A. Offer a distraction such as turning on the TV or reading a magazine

B. Inform the patient that severe pain is expected with a crush injury

C. Inform the patient that pain medication is not due for another three hours

D. Ask the patient to describe the pain in more detail

Rationale:

Correct answer: D

Unrelieved pain is a complication after a crush injury and is a sign of compartment syndrome, the result of excessive pressure built up in an enclosed muscle space, usually due to bleeding or swelling after injury. This excessive pressure impacts blood flow into and out of the affected tissue and requires fasciotomy surgery to release the pressure and prevent permanent injury.

The nurse should gather more assessment data, such as asking the patient to describe the pain in more detail. The nurse should also assess for color, pulse, and sensation and call the healthcare provider. Compartment syndrome is a medical emergency that can cause irreversible neuromuscular damage if the pressure is not released within 4-6 hours.

A is incorrect because this dismisses the problem. The nurse must investigate the unrelieved pain

B is incorrect because it is the nurse's responsibility to assess further rather than waiting three hours.

C is incorrect because if compartment syndrome is ruled out, the nurse should advocate for more or stronger pain medication.

Select All That Apply

73. A patient is placed on isolation precautions for methicillin resistant staphylococcus aureus (MRSA) infection. The nurse knows the factors to be considered when providing care include (Select all that apply):
    A. The patient's need for social interaction
    B. Isolation type required
    C. Cultural background of the patient
    D. Organizing care to minimize transporting the patient out of the room
    E. E. How the infection was contracted

Rationale:

Correct answer: A, B, C, D

Patients in isolation are at risk for depression, loneliness, and sensory deprivation. Social interaction is necessary with staff and visitors, as long as personal protective equipment (PPE) is worn. The nurse needs to know which isolation type is required for MRSA to safely care for this patient. Cultural background is important to help the nurse know how to communicate with the patient therapeutically.

Patients in isolation should stay confined to their hospital room for the duration of their isolation, if possible. If it is necessary to transport the patient to another part of the healthcare facility for a test or procedure, precautions must be followed during transport and within procedure rooms. MRSA requires contact isolation with the use of gown and gloves to prevent spread.

E is incorrect because knowledge of how the infection was contracted does not affect how nursing care will be delivered.

74. The nurse on the intensive care unit is caring for intubated patients. The nurse knows that which of the following interventions can prevent ventilator-associated pneumonia (VAP)? (Select all that apply):

    A. Elevating the head of the bed at 15 degrees
    B. Repositioning the patient every two hours
    C. Providing oral care with chlorhexidine every eight hours
    D. Maintaining cuff pressure at 30 cm H_2O to prevent secretions from entering lower airways
    E. Institute weaning trials

Rationale:

Correct answer: B, C, E

VAP is a lung infection that develops after a patient has been intubated for more than 24 hours. This can be prevented by keeping the patient's head elevated greater than 30 degrees, performing routine oral care, cleansing the oral cavity with chlorhexidine at least every eight hours, and performing endotracheal suctioning. The nurse works with the respiratory therapist to initiate weaning trials to determine if the patient is progressing towards the goal of becoming extubated.

A is incorrect because the head of the bed should be kept elevated at least 30 degrees.

D is incorrect because cuff pressures should be maintained less than 25cm H_2O (14-20 mm Hg) and should generally be checked every eight hours. Tissue necrosis can be caused by high tracheostomy cuff pressure over a prolonged period of time.

75. The nurse is preparing to irrigate a patient's wound. The nurse knows which of the following reduces risk for infection during irrigation? (Select all that apply):

    A. Use sterile technique
    B. The patient is positioned so the solution runs from the upper end of the wound downward.
    C. Warm irrigation solution to 98.6°F
    D. Clean the suture line after wound is irrigated
    E. Use intermittent pressure while irrigating

Rationale:

Correct answer: A, B

Wound irrigation is the steady flow of solution across a wound surface to clean out drainage, remove deeper debris or foreign materials, and cleanse the wound of microorganisms that can contribute to infection. When irrigating a wound, sterile technique and positioning the patient so the solution runs from the upper end of the wound downward will help reduce risk for infection.

C is incorrect because the irrigation solution does not need to be warmed to body temperature. Typically, room temperature sterile saline is used. Sterile water can be used if sterile saline is not available. Povidone iodine and hydrogen peroxide are sometimes indicated for irrigation of infected wounds.

D is incorrect because suture lines do not require irrigation. Irrigation is used for open wounds.

E is incorrect because slow, gentle, continuous pressure is used to irrigate a wound to prevent injury to the tissue.

76. The emergency room is at full capacity. How can the nurse ensure that patients and staff are safe? (Select all that apply):

    A. Leave the stretcher in the lowest position with rails down so that the patient can access the bathroom

    B. Use two identifiers before each intervention and before medication administration

    C. Attempt de-escalation strategies for patients who demonstrate aggressive behaviors

    D. Search the belongings of unaccompanied patients with altered mental status to gain essential medical information

    E. Isolate patients who have immune suppression disorders to prevent hospital-acquired infections

Rationale:

Correct answer: B, C, D

Nurses must use two identifiers per Joint Commission's National Patient Safety Goals in order to ensure patient safety. De-escalation strategies for aggressive or violent patients can prevent these individuals from harming themselves or the staff. If a patient arrives at the ER unaccompanied by family members and exhibits altered mental status, the nurse should search personal belongings for essential medical information such as medications or a medical alert card. Fall prevention interventions should also be performed, including leaving stretchers in lowest position with rails up, having the call light within reach, and isolating clients with signs and symptoms of contagious infectious disorders.

A is incorrect because leaving the stretcher side rails down may provide easy mobility for the patient but does not ensure patient or staff safety.

E is incorrect because isolating a patient with immune system suppression does not ensure patient or staff safety.

77. A patient is admitted with suspected severe sepsis. What does the nurse ensure is completed within three hours of identification of the risk of sepsis? (Select all that apply):

    A. Administer antibiotics
    B. Draw serum lactate levels
    C. Infuse vasopressors
    D. Administer oxygen is SpO_2 falls below 92%
    E. Obtain blood cultures

Rationale:

Correct answer: A, B, E

Serum lactate levels, blood cultures, and administration of antibiotics should all occur early when caring for a patient with suspected severe sepsis. Blood cultures must be drawn before antibiotics are initiated. The nurse should also anticipate early general surgery consultation for suspected acute abdomen and necrotizing infections.

C is incorrect because vasopressors should only be administered if the patient is hypotensive. The nurse cannot assume that all patients with suspected severe sepsis are hypotensive. Blood pressure should be monitored carefully and IV fluids should be infused to prevent dehydration and maintain circulating blood volume. Vasopressors are used when fluid resuscitation fails to maintain normal blood pressure.

D is incorrect because supplemental oxygen is given to all suspected sepsis patients, regardless of oxygen saturation level.

78. The student nurse is caring for patients on the medical floor. In order to transmit infection, which factors must be present? (Select all that apply):

    A. Colonization
    B. Host
    C. Mode of transmission
    D. Portal of entry
    E. Reservoir

Rationale:

Correct answer: B, C, D, E

The factors necessary for infection transmission include a host (individual who carries the pathogen), reservoir (individual susceptible to the infection), portal of entry (access into the reservoir's body), mode of transmission (ability of the pathogen to reach the reservoir from the host).

A is incorrect because colonization is not a factor in infection transmission. An individual may be colonized with bacteria, but not get sick or show signs and symptoms of infection.

79. The clinic nurse caring for patients knows which of the following statements regarding standard precautions are true? (Select all that apply):

   A. Don an isolation gown when performing hygiene on patients
   B. Sneeze into your sleeve or into a tissue that you throw away
   C. Maintain a 3-foot *safe* space from the patient who has an infection
   D. Use personal protective equipment as needed for patient care
   E. Wear gloves when touching patient excretions or secretions

Rationale:

Correct answer: D, E

Standard precautions are used when coming into contact with bodily secretions, excretions (except sweat), mucous membranes, and non-intact skin, regardless of whether infection is present or not. Gloves should always be worn when working with these materials. Other personal protective equipment (PPE) is based on care being provided.

A is incorrect because a gown is not necessary for providing hygiene on a patient with standard precautions unless the care is going to involve the splashing of bodily substances onto the clothes of the healthcare worker.

B is incorrect because sneezing into the sleeve or a tissue is respiratory etiquette, but not a component of standard precautions.

C is incorrect because safe space is not a component of standard precautions. It is unrealistic for members of the nursing team to maintain a distance of 3 feet away from patients at all times. If a patient is on droplet precautions, the gown, gloves, mask, and goggles must be worn by anyone coming within 3 feet of the infected patient.

80. The nurse is admitting a patient with suspected tuberculosis (TB) to the medical unit. Which of the following actions are best for the nurse to perform? (Select all that apply):

A. Admit the patient to a negative-airflow room

B. Maintain a distance of 3 feet from the patient, when possible

C. Order specialized masks/respirators for the healthcare staff

D. Other than wearing gloves, no special actions are needed

E. Wash hands with chlorhexidine after providing care

Rationale:

Correct answer: A, C

Patients with suspected TB are admitted to airborne precautions including negative airflow rooms and use of an N95 or PAPR mask when the nurse is providing care.

B is incorrect because the 3-foot distance applies to droplet precautions.

D incorrect because a negative airflow room and special mask must be utilized with airborne precautions.

E is incorrect because chlorhexidine is used for cleaning hands before surgery, for disinfecting surgical equipment, and for mouth care and treating oral yeast infections.

81. The nursing instructor is teaching the student nurse about infection. When the student asks why older adults are more susceptible to infection than younger adults, what reasons does the instructor give? (Select all that apply):

A. Older adults have a reduction in immune function

B. The older adult may have decreased cough and gag reflexes

C. Gastric secretions become less acidic with age

D. Older adults have an increase in lymphocytes and antibody production

E. The older adult has thinning skin that is less protective

Rationale:

Correct answer: A, B, C, E

Older adults are more susceptible to infection due to the natural decrease in immune function that occurs with older age. Decreased gag and cough reflexes are also common as adults age, potentially making it more difficult to clear secretions from the airways, increasing the risk for respiratory infections. Gastric acid helps kill bacteria that enters the GI tract.

The aging process decreases gastric juice acidity, thereby reducing the stomach's ability to kill harmful bacteria ingested on food. Thin skin and decreased lymphocytes and antibodies are also common in the elderly, decreasing skin integrity and ability of the body to fight off pathogens.

D is correct because older adults tend to have decreased lymphocytes and antibodies which are responsible for immunity and fighting off infection.

82. A 73-year-old patient is returned to the nursing unit after hip replacement surgery. The patient is disoriented and restless. Which actions can be delegated to the unlicensed assistive personnel (UAP) by the nurse? (Select all that apply):

    A. Apply an abduction pillow to the patient's legs
    B. Assess the skin under the abduction pillow straps every two hours
    C. Place pillows under the heels to keep them off the bed
    D. Monitor cognition to determine when the patient can get up out of bed
    E. Take and record vital signs per unit/facility policy

Rationale:

Correct answer: A, C, E

It is within the scope of practice of the UAP to apply an abduction pillow, elevate the patient's heels on a pillow, and take and record vital signs. Any abnormal findings should be reported to the RN immediately. The UAP can also perform standard procedures on stable patients, such as I&O, ambulating, assisting with meals (if swallowing is not impaired), bathing, encouraging incentive spirometer use, application of sequential compression devices, turning, repositioning, checking blood glucose, and assisting to the bathroom.

B is incorrect because assessment is a nursing responsibility.

D is incorrect because determining when the patient can get up is a nursing responsibility.

83. The home health nurse is visiting a client who had a hip replacement last week. The client is still using a walker with partial weight-bearing. What safety precautions should the nurse recommend? (Select all that apply):

    A. Have an elevated toilet seat installed in the home bathroom
    B. Install grab bars in the shower and near the toilet
    C. Step into the bathtub with the affected leg first
    D. Remove all throw rugs throughout the house
    E. Use a shower chair while taking a shower

Rationale:

Correct answer: A, B, D, E

An elevated toilet seat, grab bars, removal of throw rugs, and use of a shower chair are all applicable for safety for this patient. Post-hip-replacement patients may also need assistive devices for putting on socks and shoes at home. The bed should be low enough for the patient's feet to touch the floor when sitting on the side of the bed. The dressing on the surgical wound should be kept clean and dry.

C is incorrect because, with partial weight-bearing, it is unsafe for the patient to step into the bathtub with the operative side first. This might also require the patient to bend the affected hip greater than 90 degrees, which is contraindicated. The patient should be taught to use a stepstool when entering the tub or a vehicle to ensure that the affected leg does not bend more than 90 degrees.

84. The nurse is caring for a patient who sustained injury to the medulla. When assessing the patient, which clinical manifestations should be expected? (Select all that apply):

   A. Loss of smell
   B. Impaired swallowing
   C. Visual changes
   D. Inability to shrug shoulders
   E. Loss of gag reflex

Rationale:

Correct answer: B, D, E

The medulla is the origin from cranial nerves IX (glossopharyngeal), X (vagus), XI (accessory), XII (hypoglossal), VII (facial), and VIII (acoustic). Damage to these nerves will cause impaired swallowing, inability to shrug the shoulders, and loss of gag reflex. For safety, the nurse needs to monitor the patient for swallowing to prevent aspiration of food and fluids.

A is incorrect because sense of smell is affected by injury to the limbic system, not the medulla.

C is incorrect because visual changes are expected with injury to the occipital lobe of the brain, not the medulla.

85. The nurse is planning care for the patient admitted with epilepsy. Which of the following interventions should the nurse include? (Select all that apply):

   A. Prepare suction equipment at the bedside
   B. Have a padded tongue blade available at the bedside

C. Only allow clear PO fluids

D. Keep bedrails up at all times when the patient is in the bed

E. Keep the patient on strict bed-rest

F. Ensure IV access is patent

Rationale:

Correct answer: A, D, F

Suction equipment, as well as oxygen, must be available. While the patient is in bed, the bedrails should be up and padded to prevent a fall or injury. The patient should have IV access for when drug therapy is required to stop a seizure.

B is incorrect because padded tongue blades can cause injury during a seizure and shouldn't be utilized. Nothing should be inserted into the mouth during a seizure.

C is incorrect because a well-balanced diet should be ordered for the patient. If the patient has a seizure, the nurse should monitor the patient closely during the seizure and during the postictal state and not allow anything PO until the patient is alert, oriented, and stable.

E is incorrect because the patient should be encouraged to ambulate while admitted, to maintain mobility and prevent atelectasis.

86. The nurse assisted a healthcare provider in performing a lumbar puncture on a patient earlier and is reviewing lab results. Which of the following cerebrospinal fluid (CSF) lab results signify the possibility of viral meningitis? (Select all that apply):

   A. Clear

   B. Cloudy

   C. Increased protein level

   D. Normal glucose level

   E. Presence of bacterial organisms

   F. Elevated white blood cell count

Rationale:

Correct answer: A, C, D

In a patient with viral meningitis, the cerebrospinal fluid will be clear in color, have a slightly elevated protein level, and normal glucose level.

B is incorrect because viral meningitis does not cause cloudiness of cerebrospinal fluid. This is indicative of a bacterial infection.

E is incorrect because it is indicative of bacterial meningitis.

F is incorrect because it is indicative of bacterial meningitis.

87. The nurse is educating the new unlicensed assistive personnel (UAP) about safety practices on the medical-surgical unit. Which of the following actions by the UAP demonstrates correct understanding of safety? (Select all that apply):

    A.   The UAP leaves the bed in the lowest position and raises all side rails after checking vital signs
    B.   The UAP notifies the nurse immediately of an abnormal blood glucose level
    C.   The UAP leaves the call light within reach of the patient when leaving the room
    D.   The UAP uses hand sanitizer after providing care to the patient with *Clostridium difficile*
    E.   The UAP leaves a handwritten note for the nurse when a patient's blood pressure is elevated

Rationale:

Correct answer: B, C

The UAP needs to immediately notify the nurse of abnormal blood glucose levels, so this is an appropriate action. The UAP should leave the call light within reach of the patient when leaving the room, so the patient can call for help if needed. This promotes some sense of control over their environment and can reduce anxiety and feelings of abandonment related to the hospital stay.

A is incorrect because raising all side rails is a form of restraint. Least restrictive measures should be used to provide for patient safety. If all side rails are up, the patient cannot independently get out of bed. All side rails up should only be used when needed to protect a patient who may fall out of bed.

D is incorrect because when caring for a patient with *Clostridium difficile*, hands must be washed with soap and water to prevent spread of bacterial spores. *C. difficile* is not effectively killed by alcohol-based hand sanitizer.

E is incorrect because the UAP needs to immediately notify the nurse of elevated blood pressure. If a note is written, this may delay the nurse's intervention.

88. The nurse is caring for a patient who is unable to turn themselves in the bed and requires an overhead lift. The nurse knows the correct actions when using the lift include: (Select all that apply):

    A.   Have the patient propel themselves for repositioning by rocking back and forth
    B.   Leave the sling in place under the patient once seated in the chair

C. Raise the patient above the bed with the lift before laterally positioning the patient over the chair

D. Have the patient hook the sling to involve them in their care

E. Use two personnel when utilizing the sling for patient safety

Rationale:

Correct answer: B, C, E

When using a sling to lift and reposition a patient, using two personnel is required to prevent injury to the healthcare team. After transferring the patient to a chair, the sling should remain under the patient to provide for ease when returning the patient to the bed. The patient should be raised above the bed before lateral positioning to maintain patient safety.

A is incorrect because having the patient rock back and forth puts the patient at risk for injury.

D is incorrect because patients are not educated on how to utilize the lift and this may risk injury.

89. The nurse is caring for a patient who has returned from cardiac catheterization. The patient has a sheath in place. The nurse implements which of the following in the first six hours after the procedure? (Select all that apply):

    A. Remind the patient to keep the affected leg straight
    B. Remove the sheath when the patient complains of pain
    C. Check the dressing for bleeding and assess distal pulses
    D. Notify the healthcare provider if the patient has chest pain unrelieved by nitroglycerin
    E. Get the patient out of bed with the sheath in place

Rationale:

Correct answer: A, C, D

Cardiac catheterization is performed by accessing the femoral artery and using a guidewire under fluoroscopy to examine the cardiac vessels for blockage or stenosis. The sheath is sometimes left in the groin as heparin is administered to prevent blood clots around the sheath, and early discontinuation may cause excess bleeding.

The leg with the sheath should be kept straight as long as the sheath is in place and for a minimum of one hour after sheath discontinuation to prevent injury to the femoral artery. Checking the site for bleeding or swelling and assessing distal pulses is a safe practice to prevent loss of the affected extremity. Notifying the healthcare provider for chest pain unrelieved by nitroglycerin is also safe because the patient may need to return to the catheterization lab.

B is incorrect because some pain is expected, and early discontinuation of the sheath will cause excessive bleeding. It is not within the nurse's scope of practice to remove the sheath.

E is incorrect because getting the patient out of bed with the femoral sheath in place will cause damage to the femoral artery and potential loss of the affected extremity. The patient must remain on bed rest while the sheath is in place.

90. The nurse is caring for a patient who had coronary artery bypass grafting (CABG) two days ago. The patient is sitting in the chair when the nurse enters the room and finds the patient to be cold, pale, and with a decreased level of consciousness. Which of the following actions by the nurse are correct? (Select all that apply):

    A. Call the Rapid Response team
    B. Return the patient to the bed
    C. Check vital signs
    D. Administer oxygen by nasal cannula
    E. Check morning lab results

Rationale:

Correct answer: A, B, C, D, E

All of the actions are correct for this patient. The Rapid Response team will assist in care and facilitate a transfer to a higher level of care if indicated. The patient should be assisted back into the bed to prevent a fall or injury. Vital signs should be checked for hypotension. Administration of oxygen is appropriate for this patient because the symptoms indicate hypoxia. Checking morning lab results for complete blood cell count to rule out bleeding, potassium level for cardiac function and blood sugar are all appropriate.

91. The nurse is observing a student nurse preparing a sterile field for dressing change. Which of the following actions by the student nurse are correct? (Select all that apply):

    A. Dropping the inner package of sterile gloves onto the sterile field
    B. Placing the sterile drape on the bedside table and turning around to grab the package of sterile dressings behind them
    C. Keeping their hands above their waist while the sterile gloves are on
    D. Dropping the wrapped sterile dressings on the sterile drape from 6 inches above the drape
    E. Maintaining a 1-inch border around the sterile drape

Rationale:

Correct answer: A, C, E

Maintaining sterile protocol is important when performing a dressing change to prevent infection. Dropping the inner package of sterile gloves onto the sterile field is appropriate as the inner package is sterile. Keeping the sterile gloved hands above the waist is appropriate to maintain sterility of the gloves. Maintaining a 1-inch border around the sterile drape will maintain the sterility of the supplies placed on it.

B is incorrect because one should never turn their back on a sterile field.

D is incorrect because the outer package of sterile dressings is not sterile.

92. The nurse on the surgical unit has just sent a patient to surgery after administration of preoperative medication. The nurse receives a call from the surgical nurse that the consent for the surgery has not been signed. Which of the following actions should the nurse take? (Select all that apply):

    A. Notify the healthcare provider to cancel the surgery
    B. Notify the nursing supervisor
    C. Let the surgery proceed as scheduled
    D. Call for the patient to be brought back to the surgical unit
    E. Take responsibility for the lack of signed consent

Rationale:

Correct answer: B, E

The nurse who originally cared for the pre-op patient is responsible for assuring the consent has been signed before transferring the patient to the pre-op department. If the patient is transferred before the consent has been signed, the nurse should take responsibility and notify the nursing supervisor, which is following the nursing vertical chain of command. The consent must be signed by the patient before the surgery can be performed, and the patient must be informed of why the procedure is needed, as well as risks.

A is incorrect because the decision to cancel surgery will be made by the healthcare provider, and the pre-op nurse is responsible for communicating with the healthcare provider at this time. If the patient is still alert and oriented, despite pre-op medication, it may still be possible to obtain signed consent.

C is incorrect because this is out of the surgical unit nurse's control. The patient is now in the care of the pre-op nurse and signed consent must be signed before the surgery can be performed.

D is incorrect because the consent can be signed by the patient in preoperative services before general anesthesia is administered, as long as the patient is still alert, oriented, and able to verbally acknowledge understanding of the procedure and risks.

93. The nurse on the medical unit is caring for a patient who is confused and trying to climb out of the bed. Which of the following interventions by the nurse will prevent patient injury? (Select all that apply):

    A. Have a family member sit with the patient
    B. Notify the nursing supervisor
    C. Place the patient in restraints
    D. Activate the bed alarm
    E. Administer a sedative via IV push

Rationale:

Correct answer: A, B, D

A confused patient is at a higher risk for falls and injury. Several safety mechanisms should be implemented in order to prevent injury to the patient. Having a family member sit with the patient can help keep the patient-oriented and calm. The nursing supervisor should be contacted about any safety issues, and the supervisor can help with obtaining a patient sitter if another staff member (such as a UAP) or family member is unable to stay at the bedside. Activating the bed alarm can assist in quick alert of the staff when the patient is attempting to get out of bed, thus preventing injury.

C is incorrect because restraints can agitate the patient and cause injury. The nurse should attempt the less restrictive measures listed above before restraining a patient, and restraints should only be used as a last measure for keeping a patient in bed.

E is incorrect because sedatives can worsen confusion and cause injury. The nurse should attempt to provide for patient safety with non-pharmacologic measures first.

94. A patient on the medical-surgical unit is experiencing an anaphylactic-type allergic reaction to a medication. The nurse calls the rapid response team and the healthcare provider, who respond to the bedside. The healthcare provider orders epinephrine 1 mg IV. What is the correct action by the nurse? (Select all that apply):

    A. Administer the epinephrine as ordered
    B. Question the medication order
    C. Have the unlicensed assistive personnel (UAP) check vital signs, including oxygen saturation level
    D. Ask the charge nurse to review the medication reconciliation to identify the causative agent
    E. Prepare to give packed red blood cells after the epinephrine is administered

Rationale:

Correct answer: B, C, D

Anaphylaxis is a deadly allergic reaction to a causative agent that causes vascular collapse (hypotension) and swelling of the airway. Other effects include dyspnea, decreased oxygen saturation, and flushing. When a patient experiences an anaphylactic-type allergic reaction to a medication, epinephrine 1 mg is administered intramuscularly (IM) or subcutaneously.

The nurse should question the order by the healthcare provider as administration of the epinephrine IV may cause myocardial infarction. It is appropriate for the nurse to check vital signs and monitor oxygen saturation, and these tasks can be delegated to the UAP. It is also appropriate to have another member of the nursing team review the medication reconciliation to identify what caused the harmful reaction.

(Note: The primary RN should remain at the bedside caring for the patient while someone else checks the chart.)

A is incorrect because administration of epinephrine IV could cause myocardial infarction. The correct route for anaphylaxis is IM or subcutaneous. The nurse is responsible for checking the correct strength of epinephrine is given. 1:100 is only for inhalation; 1:1000 is for IM or subcutaneous administration.

E is incorrect because packed red blood cells are not often given as emergency treatment for anaphylaxis.

95. The nurse is caring for a patient admitted to the medical floor with severe acute respiratory syndrome (SARS) after traveling abroad. Which of the following personal protective equipment (PPE) does the nurse need to wear? (Select all that apply):

   A. Gloves
   B. Gown
   C. Mask
   D. Goggles or eye shield
   E. Hood and respirator

   Rationale:

   Correct answer: A, B, C, D

SARS is a disease that is not completely understood, including its transmission. Every mode of transmission is considered to be possible including airborne, droplet, and contact. The nurse should wear gloves, a gown, mask, and goggles, or an eye shield. SARS symptoms include high fever, headache, overall body aches, and most patients develop pneumonia.

E is incorrect because a hood and respirator are not necessary if all the other PPE is worn.

96. The nurse is reviewing new orders for a patient and discovers potential errors in the medications ordered. Which of the following medications are correct for the patient admitted for hypertension and unstable angina, complaining of severe chest pain? (Select all that apply):

    A. Furosemide IV
    B. Morphine IV
    C. Nitroglycerin sublingual
    D. Dopamine IV
    E. Metoprolol-XL PO

Rationale:

Correct answer: A, B, C

Hypertension (or elevated blood pressure) and unstable angina (or chest pain) that occur with or without exertion, frequently occur together. Hypertension is treated with antihypertensive medications, such as IV beta-blockers, and diuretics, such as furosemide. Unstable angina is treated with nitroglycerin, which is a vasodilator and can relieve chest pain. Morphine is given for the severe chest pain, as it can treat the pain and also decrease the work of the heart (morphine decreases preload.) The nurse has the authority *and* legal obligation to question any order that is believed to be an error, for patient safety.

D is incorrect because dopamine is administered to a patient who is hypotensive. This powerful vasoconstrictor is contraindicated in a patient experiencing hypertension, as it will only worsen the elevated BP.

E is incorrect because extended-release beta-blockers are not used for hypertension with unstable angina because the effect will be delayed. For quick relief of hypertension, metoprolol should be given IV. Metoprolol-XL is used as a daily dose to control hypertension in stable patients.

97. The emergency room nurse is caring for a 24-year-old patient who came in with her husband who reports she fell down the stairs. The patient has multiple bruises at different stages of healing, a black

eye, and a splint on the right wrist. She avoids making eye contact, and the husband answers most of the questions. Which of the following actions by the nurse are appropriate? (Select all that apply):

A. Accompany the patient privately to the bathroom to provide a urine sample
B. Notify the police that abuse is suspected
C. Notify the charge nurse of suspected abuse
D. Ask the patient and her husband about details of the fall
E. Walk the patient through the department where brochures about domestic violence services are visible

Rationale:

Correct answer: A, C, E

When abuse is suspected, it is important to encourage the patient to talk about the abuse. This can be achieved by getting the patient away from the abuser, such as taking her to the bathroom for a urine sample. Notifying the charge nurse is necessary with any form of suspected abuse (domestic violence, child abuse, sexual abuse, elder abuse). The charge nurse can help with identifying safe next steps when caring for the patient and reporting further up the chain of command. Brochures about domestic violence services should be visible to all patients and taking the patient for a walk where these can be seen is extremely helpful to the patient.

B is incorrect because this type of abuse is not required to be reported. When an adult patient is the victim of potential abuse, the patient has the right to make the choice about whether authorities are to be contacted. Note: Abuse of a minor must be reported with or without the patient's approval.

D is incorrect because the patient is unlikely to give details with the abuser present, and the abuser is likely to give a false report.

98. The nurse on the medical-surgical floor has just received the shift report. According to the report, one of the patients needs to be monitored for signs and symptoms of thyroid storm. The nurse will observe the patient for which of the following? (Select all that apply):

A. Increased urine output
B. Hyperkinesis
C. Fever
D. Enlarged thyroid gland
E. Hypertension
F. Vomiting

Rationale:

Correct answer: B, C, E, F

Thyroid storm (or thyrotoxic crisis), is a state of severe hyperthyroidism. It is identified by the symptoms of hyperkinesis (increased muscle activity or overactive restlessness), tachycardia, elevated temperature, increased blood pressure, vomiting, restlessness, and coma.

A is incorrect because increased urine output is not a symptom of thyroid storm.

D is incorrect because an enlarged thyroid gland is not a symptom of thyroid storm.

99. A patient is admitted to the cardiac ICU for an acute myocardial infarction. The nurse is reviewing the patient's orders from the healthcare provider. Which of the following interventions by the nurse are appropriate? (Select all that apply):

   A. Initiate thrombolytic therapy
   B. Give the patient water to drink
   C. Oxygen at 2L via nasal cannula
   D. Monitor the patient's cardiac rhythm
   E. Encourage the patient to ambulate

Rationale:

Correct answer: A, B, C, D

During a myocardial infarction, a thrombolytic medication is administered to break down clots in the cardiac vasculature which contribute to blockage and infarction. Water is appropriate for the patient to drink in small amounts as long as the nurse monitors for fluid overload. Fluid intake should be limited to 2,000 mL daily, as too much fluid can precipitate CHF. Oxygen is beneficial to the heart during myocardial infarction. Placing the cardiac monitor is extremely important for the nurse to monitor the electrocardiogram for dysrhythmias.

E is incorrect, because during a myocardial infarction, the patient needs to rest and decrease the demand on the heart. Bed rest decreases stress on the heart and the patient should be kept in semi-fowler's position.

CHAPTER 4:

NCLEX-RN – FUNDAMENTALS: LEADERSHIP AND MANAGEMENT

Multiple Choice

1. The healthcare provider has asked the nurse to discontinue a feeding tube for an unresponsive patient based on the family's request. The nurse knows the legal basis of this order and first reviews the patient's medical record for documentation of which of the following?

   A. Court approval for discontinuation of treatment
   B. Approval by the ethics committee of the facility
   C. Healthcare provider's order for feeding tube removal
   D. Family authorization for discontinuation of treatment

Rationale:

Correct answer: D

An appointed family member or legal guardian has the authority to make decisions for a patient who is incompetent or unable to make decisions for themselves. Withholding and withdrawal of life support is a process through which various medical interventions are either not given to patients or removed from them with the expectation that the patients will die from their underlying illnesses.

The healthcare provider writes the order to discontinue treatment once the decision is made. This is usually a collaborative decision including the healthcare provider(s), healthcare workers, and family members. The nurse's main priority is ensuring that the family has signed authorization for the discontinuation of treatment.

A is incorrect because a court order is only necessary for certain circumstances.

B is incorrect because some facilities may require ethics committee involvement, but this is not the nurse's first action.

C is incorrect because although the written order by the healthcare provider is necessary, it is not the nurse's first action.

2. The nurse on the rehabilitation is planning a multidisciplinary research project examining the effects of immobility on patients' stress levels. Which of the following is the most important principle in the planning phase of the research project?

    A. Patients have the right to refuse participation
    B. Collaboration with other healthcare disciplines is essential to nursing practice success
    C. On-staff healthcare providers must cooperate for project success
    D. Nurse executive consultation must be completed due to the length of the research process

Rationale:

Correct answer: A

This research project includes human subjects, so ethically and legally, the patients retain the right to refuse to participate in the research.

B is incorrect because although other healthcare disciplines may be considered in the project, this is not the most important principle.

C is incorrect because although cooperation of healthcare providers must be considered, this is not the most important principle. Providing privacy and autonomy for patients to make their own decisions is most important.

D is incorrect because although the nurse executive may be consulted, this is not the most important principle. The nurse on the rehab unit must have permission from the nursing manager to complete a research project. The nurse manager is responsible for handling interactions with the executive nursing team, if necessary.

3. The nurse manager of the inpatient unit identifies an issue and holds a meeting for all shifts. An analysis of the issue, along with proposals for action is presented, and the team members are invited to participate with comments and ideas. What type of leadership does this nurse manager demonstrate?

    A. Situational
    B. Laissez-faire
    C. Participative
    D. Authoritarian

Rationale:

Correct answer: C

This nurse manager is demonstrating participative leadership, which is between authoritarian and democratic styles. The participative leader presents analyses of issues and proposals for solving, with input from the staff. Once comments and input have been collected and analyzed, the leader makes the decision.

A is incorrect because the situational leader adapts their leadership style depending on events and situations. Situational leaders often move between other leadership styles, according to the needs of the organization.

B is incorrect because the laissez-faire leader gives up leadership and responsibility and allows the staff to work without supervision or direction. The idea behind this leadership style is to do what you want as long as you get the job done right. From a laissez-faire leader's perspective, the key to success is to build a strong team, and then stay out of the way.

D is incorrect because the authoritarian leader focuses on tasks and directives. The authoritative leadership style involves a leader making decisions on policies, procedures, and group objectives with little or no input from their team members or followers.

4. The charge nurse on the telemetry unit notices that a staff nurse is unable to reasonably meet patient needs in a timely manner, problem solve, and prioritize patient care. The responsibility of the charge nurse is to:

   A. Supervise this staff nurse closely for task completion
   B. Ask staff members to assist this staff nurse in completing work
   C. Provide support to this staff nurse and identify underlying causes of the issue
   D. Report this staff nurse to the supervisor to resolve the issue

Rationale:

Correct answer: C

Fundamental charge nurse responsibilities include planning, coordinating, and evaluating unit nursing activities. When monitoring the quality of patient care being delivered by other nursing staff members, the charge nurse implements measures to correct inadequacies noted in the quality of patient care administered on the unit. Safe patient care is the goal. Safe care can be delivered when the charge nurse attempts to identify and improve underlying issues that are challenging the success of the staff nurse.

A is incorrect because it does not help the staff nurse provide safe patient care.

B is incorrect because it shifts the burden to the other nurses and staff on the unit. This action may prevent the others from providing safe care to the patients assigned to them.

D is incorrect because it is a punitive action.

5. The new nurse graduate is organizing patient assignments and tasks for the shift under the observation of the nurse preceptor. The nurse preceptor should intervene if the new nurse graduate does what?

    A. Provides time for the unexpected

    B. Lists supplies for a task

    C. Prioritizes patient needs and tasks

    D. Plans documentation for the end of the shift

Rationale:

Correct answer: D

Documentation should be completed throughout the shift and when tasks and interventions are performed. This provides for better recall and more accurate documentation in the legal patient record. Charting as the shift progresses also helps keep documentation at the end of the shift to a more manageable load. Patient improvement or decline is easier to spot when events are charted in the order they occur. Waiting until the end of shift to record assessments, may lead to inadvertent omission of important patient details. If documentation will be delayed, the nurse should keep a list of notes throughout the shift to expand on when charting later.

(Note: The nurse should also avoid documenting in advance of care provided. This practice is illegal falsification of the record, contributes to errors and confusion, and can pose a threat to patient safety.)

A is incorrect because it is part of effective time management. If the nurse leaves time in the day for the unexpected, this helps with flexibility when unpredictable events occur while caring for patients. At the start of the shift, it's important for the nurse to get a feel for the pace at which things have been going on in the unit. Consider: general acuity level of patients, who may be able to help if the nurse gets overwhelmed, what treatments and procedures are planned for the day?

B is incorrect because it is part of effective time management. Before beginning a task, the nurse should list and collect all supplies needed.

C is incorrect because it is part of effective time management. The nurse should have a plan for the day that includes assessments, patient meals, medication administration, time-specific procedures/activities, patients who may need extra time for teaching, and ADLs. Plan time for charting at least three times during shift and chart any PRN meds immediately. Review the schedule every two hours to make adjustments for changes.

6. The nurse is working with a nursing student caring for a patient admitted for cerebrovascular accident with unilateral weakness. The nurse intervenes when the student does which of the following?

    A. Tells the patient to survey the environment
    B. Approaches the patient from the unaffected side
    C. Places the bedside table and personal objects on the affected side
    D. Moves the bedside commode and chair to the affected side

Rationale:

Correct answer: B

The goal of care for a patient with a stroke and unilateral weakness is to focus attention on the patient's affected side, as a stroke can cause neglect and unawareness to that side. This increases the patient's risk for injury. The nurse should approach the patient so that they have to turn their head toward the injured side, which promotes eye contact.

A is incorrect because the patient should survey the environment to increase awareness of potential risks. This promotes patient safety and reduces risk for falls.

C is incorrect because the bedside table and personal objects should be placed on the affected side. Additionally, the TV should be positioned so the patient has to turn their head to the affected side when watching.

D is incorrect because the bedside commode and chair should be moved to the affected side. The room should be arranged to maximize stimulation of the affected side.

7. The nursing instructor asks the students to define critical pathways. Which student statement indicates further instruction is needed?

    A. Critical pathways are developed collaboratively and with multidisciplinary members of the healthcare team.
    B. Critical pathways provide the most effective way of monitoring care and reducing length of stay for the patient.
    C. Critical pathways are based on appropriate standards of patient care.
    D. Critical pathways are nursing care plans developed using steps of the nursing process.

Rationale:

Correct answer: D

Critical pathways are different from nursing care plans. A critical pathway is a set of concurrent actions performed in a certain order to achieve a goal in optimizing care and outcomes for patients. These are not based solely on nursing and require the multidisciplinary healthcare team.

A is incorrect because it is an accurate definition of critical pathways.

B is incorrect because it is an accurate definition of critical pathways.

C is incorrect because it is an accurate definition of critical pathways.

8. The community health nurse is working with a local disaster relief effort following a hurricane. The community goals are to prevent injury and death, find shelter for survivors, and to provide support, counseling, and medical care. Which type of prevention is described here?

    A. Primary
    B. Secondary
    C. Tertiary
    D. Aggregate care

Rationale:

Correct answer: C

Tertiary prevention is classified by reduction of disability, injury, and damage after a crisis.

A is incorrect because primary prevention involves the steps taken to prevent a crisis from occurring.

B is incorrect because secondary prevention involves taking actions during an event to reduce the intensity and duration of the crisis. The community health nurse above is working after the hurricane, not during the event.

D is incorrect because there is no aggregate care prevention.

9. The nurse manager is planning to change the nursing unit care delivery from team to primary nursing. Staff resistance to the change is expected. Which primary technique should the nurse manager use to implement the change?

    A. Gradually introduce the change
    B. Confront those involved in the process of change
    C. Coerce the staff to change implementation
    D. Manipulate participants during the process of change

Rationale:

Correct answer: A

When change is resisted, the primary technique that should be used to implement change is a gradual introduction. This will slowly introduce the change to the staff, giving them time to adapt, and can decrease the amount of potential resistance.

B is incorrect because when resistance occurs, confrontation is used to help articulate the need for the change. A gradual introduction to the change can prevent the resistance, eliminating the need for confrontation.

C is incorrect because coercion is ineffective for helping staff members embrace changes in the workplace.

D is incorrect because manipulation is covert, and vital information may be left out and perceived negatively by participants. This also is not the most successful method for change implementation.

10. The nurse is preparing for the admission of a patient who will have an internal cervical radiation device implanted. Which of the following interventions does the nurse implement for this patient?

    A. Prepare the private room at the end of the hallway
    B. Hang a door sign that limits visitation to one hour
    C. Assign one nurse to care for the patient during her stay to promote continuity of care.
    D. Place a dirty linen cart outside the room for dirty linens

Rationale:

Correct answer: A

A patient who receives an internal cervical radiation implant should be in a private room that decreases the risk of exposure of radiation to others. A sign should be placed indicating the presence of radiation for safety.

B is incorrect because visitors must be educated about the need to limit close contact with the patient to no more than 30 minutes. Visitors can wear a dosimeter device, which will sound an alarm when they have reached their 30-minute exposure limit. Then, they can remain in the room for longer as long as they remain more than 3 feet away from the patient. This is done to prevent visitors from overexposure to radiation.

C is incorrect because nurses should be rotated in caring for the patient to decrease exposure to the radiation. Each member of the nursing team assigned to this patient will wear a dosimeter and change assignments after 30 minutes of exposure has been met. One is only exposed when within close contact with the patient. Patient care should be clustered to limit the amount of time spent close to the patient/bed.

D is incorrect because a dedicated dirty linen cart should be placed inside the room so that if the implant becomes displaced, it can be located in the dirty linen cart.

11. The nurse is working with a nursing student to care for a patient who had a chest tube with drainage system placed for pneumothorax yesterday. The nurse intervenes if the nursing student includes which of the following in the plan of care for the patient?

    A. Position the patient in semi-fowler's position
    B. Add water to the suction control chamber to maintain 20 cm H_2O
    C. Tape connection sites to prevent disconnection
    D. Instruct patient to avoid deep breathing and coughing

Rationale:

Correct answer: D

Deep breathing and coughing are important for any patient who has a chest tube to prevent atelectasis and pneumonia and assist in lung re-expansion. The nurse should teach the patient to change position frequently. The drainage system must be maintained below the level of insertion with no kinks in the tubing.

A is incorrect because semi-fowler's position facilitates breathing with a chest tube in place.

B is incorrect because maintaining the water level in the suction chamber is appropriate for maintaining the suction level.

C is incorrect because the connections between chest tube and drainage system should be taped to prevent disconnection. If the chest tube becomes dislodged from the patient, the nurse should cover the site with a sterile dressing tented on one side to allow for escape of air. If the tubing becomes disconnected from the device, the contaminated tip should be cut off, then reattach with a sterile connector or immerse the tip into sterile water until the system can be re-established.

12. The nurse is planning care for a patient who just had a cast applied to the left lower extremity. The nurse instructs the licensed practical nurse (LPN/LVN) caring for the patient to do which of the following to prevent compartment syndrome?

    A. Elevate the left lower extremity and apply ice
    B. Elevate the left lower extremity and cover with blankets
    C. Place the left lower extremity in a dependent position and apply ice
    D. Maintain the left lower extremity horizontally and apply ice

Rationale:

Correct answer: A

Compartment syndrome is caused when edema occurs where trauma was sustained, causing swelling in the intravascular space that must be relieved with fasciotomy. The nurse should direct the LPN to elevate the left lower extremity and apply ice to control edema.

B is incorrect because blankets will not prevent edema. The extremity should be assessed frequently for signs of compartment syndrome: paralysis, pulselessness, pallor, pain, and paresthesia.

C is incorrect because a dependent position will cause edema.

D is incorrect because keeping the affected extremity horizontal will not prevent edema. Elevation is necessary to reduce blood flow to the affected limb and prevent edema.

13. The charge nurse is making rounds on all restrained patients for quality control and patient safety. Which observation requires the charge nurse to immediately contact the assigned nurse?

    A. Safety knot utilized to secure a soft wrist restraint
    B. A patient's chart indicates a vest restraint is released every two hours
    C. A vest restraint is applied very tightly
    D. Call light within reach of a patient with soft wrist restraints

Rationale:

Correct answer: C

Any type of restraint that is applied tightly can impair circulation. A vest restraint that is applied tightly can also impair breathing or cause choking as the patient moves in the bed or the chair. Restraints are used to protect patients from injury; they should not pose a risk.

A is incorrect because safety knots are used for quick release in case of emergency. Double knots are contraindicated as they can be difficult to untie.

B is incorrect because restraints must be released every two hours for skin assessment and circulation.

D is incorrect because the call light must always be within reach for a retrained patient. Similarly, the bedside table and other necessary items such as drink of water or urinal should be within reach.

14. The nurse manager is reviewing restraints with the staff. When asking about indications for restraints, which statement indicates more education is necessary?

    A. "A restraint can be applied to limit the movement of an extremity."

B. "Restraints can be applied to keep a patient in the bed at night."

C. "Restraints can prevent a violent patient from hurting themselves and the staff."

D. "Restraints can be applied to prevent the patient from pulling out invasive lines."

Rationale:

Correct answer: B

Restraints should not be applied for the purpose of preventing a patient from getting out of bed at night. Other less restrictive measures, such as bed alarms, side rails, or a sitter should be used. Restraints must never be used as coercion, punishment, staff convenience, or discipline.

A is incorrect because restraints can be applied to immobilize an extremity, such as when a femoral sheath is in place or when a patient needs to keep the arm straight due to an IV at the cubital fossa of the elbow.

C is incorrect because restraints are used to prevent a patient from hurting themselves and others.

D is incorrect because restraints are used to prevent removal of invasive lines and protective dressings.

15. The nurse in the clinic wants to create a diabetic teaching program for patients. In order to meet patient needs, the first action the clinic nurse must perform is:

   A. Assess functional abilities of the patients
   B. Contact insurance companies to ensure coverage for the program
   C. Discuss the program with the multidisciplinary team
   D. Include all clinic patients in teaching sessions

Rationale:

Correct answer: A

Clinics are focused on disease prevention as well as health promotion and maintenance. The nurse must assess the patients' functional abilities and needs before creating a teaching program in order for it to be effective for the patient population. First, the nurse determines which patients are a good fit for the teaching program.

B is incorrect because insurance coverage is not assessed until patient ability and interest in participation have been established.

C is incorrect because discussing the program with the multidisciplinary team does not focus on patients' needs. The nurse should initially focus on the patients and determine who is eligible for participation and assess their interest.

D is incorrect because not all clinic patients necessarily have diabetes.

16. The RN on the surgical unit cares for a patient who complains of pain persisting after prescribed opioid analgesics have been administered by the LPN. Which of the following actions is most appropriate for the registered nurse to take?

    A. Change the LPN assignment to patients who do not have opioids ordered
    B. Notify the healthcare provider to request an increase in opioid dosage
    C. Review the patient's medication administration record (MAR) and discuss with the nursing supervisor
    D. Ask the LPN about the patient's pain control issues

Rationale:

Correct answer: C

The RN must confirm suspicion with documentation in the patient's medical record, otherwise, it is just suspicion. Every facility has policies and procedures regarding opioid use that must be followed, as well as state and federal labor laws and opioid regulations. Following the chain of command once the data is confirmed is the most appropriate choice.

A is incorrect because changing the LPN's assignment is ignoring the issue of potential substance abuse. Any form of suspected abuse should be reported to the nursing supervisor.

B is incorrect because the nurse does not have enough data at this time to determine the patient needs increased opioid dosage.

D is incorrect because confronting the LPN would not be beneficial to either party and could result in argument.

17. The nurse manager is reviewing critical pathways of patients on the medical-surgical unit. The manager has met with each nurse and performs a variance analysis on patient care. Which of the following patient scenarios indicates the manager needs to further analyze and intervene?

    A. Patient changing their own colostomy bag
    B. Purulent drainage noted from a patient's operative incision
    C. Patient who had surgery yesterday has a temp of 98.9° F
    D. Patient with newly diagnosed diabetes prepares self-injection of insulin

Rationale:

Correct answer: B

A variance is either a positive or negative deviation from critical pathways, which can delay discharge (negative variance) or speed it up (positive variance). Purulent drainage from an operative incision indicates infection, which is a negative variance and requires intervention.

A is incorrect because a patient changing their own colostomy bag is a good outcome. The nurse should encourage independence through teaching and demonstration.

C is incorrect because a normal temperature is expected. (Even a slightly elevated temperature one-day post-op is common due to the inflammatory response after surgery.)

D is incorrect because diabetes is a chronic disease and a nursing goal is for the patient to learn to care for themselves. The patient's ability to prepare their own insulin injection is good outcome, indicating patient understanding of diabetes management.

18. The nurse manager has decided to change the mode of delivery of care from team nursing to primary nursing without input from the staff. Which type of leadership style does this nurse manager demonstrate?

   A. Autocratic
   B. Situational
   C. Democratic
   D. Laissez-faire

Rationale:

Correct answer: A

An autocratic leader is task-oriented and directive. This type of leader uses the position of power to make policy and procedure decisions for the organization without input from staff.

B is incorrect because the situational leader is adaptable, moving between other leadership styles, according to the needs of the organization. Situations and events determine the style of leadership that is selected.

C is incorrect because democratic leadership empowers staff and allows input in the decision-making process.

D is incorrect because a Laissez-faire leader gives up leadership and responsibility and allows the staff to work without supervision or direction.

19. The new graduate nurse working on the medical-surgical nurse tells the nurse preceptor that participation in quality improvement (QI) is impossible because of inexperience. What is the best response by the nurse preceptor?

    A. "All nurses participate in QI at this facility."
    B. "Even though you are inexperienced, you can assist in implementing activities that improve delivery of care."
    C. "Identifying factors used to measure quality is easy."
    D. "You should join the research and quality committee."

Rationale:

Correct answer: B

It is possible for inexperienced nurses to assist in and implement QI measures and the nurse preceptor should reassure the new graduate nurse of this. Often, new graduate nurses are more up-to-date on EBP having just completed nursing school, and their knowledge is important in contributing to QI.

A is incorrect because this is a simple, dismissive statement that does not help the new nurse understand how participation is possible. It may be a true statement, but it does not address the new nurse's feelings of inexperience.

C is incorrect because identifying factors for measuring quality is not easy and is not optimal for suggesting a starting place for the new nurse. This statement is dismissive and may provide false reassurance.

D is incorrect because joining research and quality does not assist the nurse in implementing QI in daily care provision.

20. The charge nurse of the medical-surgical unit is aware that nurse drug and alcohol abuse warrants disciplinary action by the board of nursing. When working with a nurse who uses drugs or alcohol, the charge nurse knows the priority when assessing an impaired nurse is:

    A. Illegal activities related to substance abuse
    B. Physiological impact of substance abuse on the nurse's practice
    C. Whether falsification of patient records is occurring
    D. Impact of substance diversion over time

Rationale:

Correct answer: B

The charge nurse must ensure the nurse is able to provide safe, quality patient care. The impact of the substance abuse on the nurse's ability to carry out job duties is the priority.

A is incorrect because illegal activities will be addressed when the investigation is performed. Patient care is the priority.

C is incorrect because falsification of patient records will be addressed when the investigation is performed.

D is incorrect because substance diversion is the transfer of a legally prescribed controlled substance from the individual for whom it was prescribed to another individual for illicit use. The impact of substance diversion will be addressed when the investigation is performed.

21. The nurse manager has found many problems with the current patient documentation system and determines a change must be made. The first step the nurse manager should take when planning a change to the patient documentation system is:

    A. Plan strategies for implementation
    B. Evaluate goals and priorities
    C. Identify the specific problem
    D. Identify potential solutions

Rationale:

Correct answer: C

Before implementing a change, the nurse manager must gather assessment data to identify and define the specific problem. Prematurely initiating changes without appropriate identification of the problem can lengthen the change process and lead to ineffective change.

A is incorrect because planning strategies for implementation cannot be done until the actual problem has been identified.

B is incorrect because goals and priorities cannot be set or evaluated until the actual problem has been identified.

D is incorrect because identifying potential solutions will be done after the problem has been identified and the goals for change have been set.

22. The ICU nurse receives the report for a patient being admitted from the emergency department and learns the patient has been defibrillated twice for ventricular tachycardia. When preparing the patient room, which of the following items does the nurse instruct the unlicensed assistive personnel (UAP) to place at the bedside?

A. Tracheostomy set and oxygen

B. Endotracheal tube and an airway

C. Defibrillator cart

D. Cooling blanket

Rationale:

Correct answer: C

This patient has already been defibrillated twice for ventricular tachycardia, so the nurse should direct the UAP to place the defibrillator cart at the bedside to be prepared in case the patient experiences the arrhythmia when admitted to the ICU. This will save precious time versus waiting for the patient to experience the arrhythmia and running down the hall to retrieve the cart while chest compressions are performed.

A is incorrect because a tracheostomy is not indicated. If the patient's airway becomes compromised, the nurse will provide breaths using a bag-mask. If an artificial airway is needed, the patient will be orally intubated before a tracheostomy procedure is performed.

B is incorrect because, although the patient may need to be intubated if cardiac arrest occurs again, an endotracheal tube and airway is not priority and is usually found on the defibrillator cart.

D is incorrect because a cooling blanket is not indicated for this patient. No information is given about the patient's temperature trends.

23. The nurse is planning care for a patient with acute pancreatitis. Which of the following actions does the nurse instruct the unlicensed assistive personnel (UAP) to do when caring for the patient?

    A. Ambulate the patient frequently

    B. Encourage a diet high in protein

    C. Check blood glucose levels every hour

    D. Assess the patient for pain

Rationale:

Correct answer: C

Pancreatitis is characterized by inflammation due to digestive enzymes within the pancreas being activated before exiting the pancreas. It is a painful condition that can cause bleeding, tissue damage, and infection. The nurse will instruct the UAP to check the patient's blood glucose levels every hour as hyperglycemia is expected and an insulin infusion is often administered. Antibiotics, histamine-blockers, opioids, and proton-pump inhibitors will also be used. Fluid/electrolyte balance and respiratory status must also be monitored closely by the nurse.

A is incorrect because the patient will most likely be on strict bed rest.

B is incorrect because the patient will be NPO (nothing by mouth). The patient requires gastric decompression and will likely have a NG in place, attached to intermittent suction. Parenteral nutrition is often indicated for the patient with acute pancreatitis. PN allows the gut to rest.

D is incorrect because the UAP cannot perform a pain assessment. The UAP must notify the nurse if the patient complains of pain.

24. The medical-surgical nurse is observing the dialysis nurse performing hemodialysis on a patient. The dialysis nurse is drinking coffee and eating a muffin next to the dialysis machine while conversing with the patient about weekend plans. Which action by the medical-surgical nurse is best?

    A. Get some coffee and join in on the conversation
    B. Ask the patient if they would like some coffee or a muffin
    C. Observe the relationship between the patient and the dialysis nurse
    D. Ask the dialysis nurse not to eat and drink in the patient's room

Rationale:

Correct answer: D

Due to infection control purposes and standard precautions, the nurse should ask the dialysis nurse not to eat and drink in the patient's room and around the dialysis equipment.

A is incorrect because food and drink should generally not be consumed in the patient room or around dialysis equipment.

B is incorrect because eating during dialysis is generally contraindicated. If the patient needs a nutritional supplement during dialysis, foods that are small in quantity and easy to eat are recommended: nutritional supplement drinks, low-potassium fruits, and vegetables (apple, pears, peaches, celery, carrot, cucumber), or graham crackers.

(Note: coffee contains caffeine, which is a natural diuretic. During hemodialysis, fluid-volume balance must be maintained, so caffeinated beverages are contraindicated.)

C is incorrect because the nurse needs to intervene. Staff should be counseled against eating and drinking around the dialysis equipment for infection control purposes.

25. A float nurse from the medical-surgical unit has come to work on the intensive care unit (ICU). The ICU charge nurse should assign which patient to the medical-surgical nurse?

    A. Post-operative patient who had a kidney transplant four hours ago

    B. Patient who experienced cardiac arrest, on a ventilator with several IV medications infusing

    C. Patient who had coronary artery bypass grafting (CABG) two days ago

    D. Patient admitted for heart failure exacerbation with dopamine infusing

Rationale:

Correct answer: C

The medical-surgical nurse is capable of caring for stable patients. The ICU charge nurse should assign the medical-surgical nurse the most stable patients on the unit. Generally, ventilators and IV vasopressors are not customarily used on the med-surg unit. Thus, the float nurse may not be proficient in administering care for these types of patients.

A is incorrect because the medical-surgical nurse has not necessarily been trained on transplant patients. Complications after a kidney transplant include rejection, infections, post-transplant lymphoproliferative disorder, and electrolytic imbalance. The nurse should be able to apply in-depth knowledge of organ transplantation to care for the transplant patient. Analysis of the biological, psychological, and sociological effects of transplantation is necessary.

B is incorrect because the medical-surgical nurse may not be trained on ventilators or IV infusions common for this type of patient.

D is incorrect because the medical-surgical nurse may not have experience with dopamine infusions. Dopamine is a powerful vasopressor, requiring BP monitoring, peripheral pulses, and urinary output. Adverse effects include tachycardia, chest pain, and dysrhythmias. Infusion pump must be used, and headache is an early sign of drug excess.

26. The charge nurse has assisted the night shift nurse in completing the incident report for a patient who fell earlier in the shift. Once the report is completed, the charge nurse intervenes when the nurse performs which of the following?

    A. Notifies the nursing supervisor

    B. Asks the unit secretary to call the healthcare provider

    C. Documents in the patient's chart that the incident report was completed

    D. Forwards the incident report to risk management

Rationale:

Correct answer: C

It is necessary to complete an incident report following facility policy after a patient fall, but it is never documented in the patient's chart that an incident report was filed. The staff member who discovers the incident, or the one who knows the most about it, is responsible for filing the report by the end of the shift in which the event occurred. In the event of a serious error, if a nurse fails to file an incident report, the nurse may be more likely to face disciplinary action. Incident reports are a safeguard for the patients, the healthcare workers, and the entire facility.

A is incorrect because the nursing supervisor should be notified (per facility policy) when an incident report will be filed.

B is incorrect because the healthcare provider should be notified verbally. (The incident report is a higher priority than notifying the healthcare provider, though.)

D is incorrect because incident reports are sent to risk management (as well as quality assurance and insurance representatives). These groups use incident reports to track trends and to identify needed changes. Changes are implemented (policy revision, new systems implemented) to prevent similar events from happening in the future.

27. The healthcare provider is on the intensive care unit (ICU) rounding on patients when they are paged off the unit. The healthcare provider tells the nurse to write an order for Digoxin 125 mg PO daily. What is the most appropriate action by the nurse?

    A. Write the order
    B. Notify the nursing supervisor to write the order
    C. Inform the patient of the medication order
    D. Ask the healthcare provider to return to write the requested order

Rationale:

Correct answer: D

Due to the risk of errors, nurses are not to accept verbal orders from healthcare providers except in emergencies. The nurse should ask the healthcare provider to return to the unit when they are able to write the order.

A is incorrect because of the risk of medication error. (Digoxin ordered PO daily is not given for emergency heart failure patients.)

B is incorrect because of the risk of medication error, and it is inappropriate to ask someone else to write the order. The nurse can accept a verbal order for emergency situations or when the healthcare provider is outside of the hospital facility (phone order). If the nurse is going to accept a verbal order, the nurse personally must write the order for the healthcare provider to sign later. The nurse cannot re-delegate to anyone in the nursing team to write the verbal order. Notifying the nurse supervisor is not a necessary component of accepting a verbal order.

C is incorrect because although the patient should be informed of the medication order, it is not the most appropriate action.

28. The nurse on the medical-surgical unit receives a report from the emergency room on a patient placed in skeletal leg traction of the left leg. When preparing the room for the patient, which of the following items does the nurse ask the unlicensed assistive personnel (UAP) to place in the room?

   A. Antibiotic ointment
   B. Bilateral sequential compression devices
   C. Bed trapeze
   D. Cold therapy system

Rationale:

Correct answer: C

A bed trapeze is a lifting assistant that is placed over the bed to help patients lift and reposition themselves in the bed. A bed trapeze is essential for this patient to prevent extra traction from being placed on the extremity which could compromise healing and alignment of the bones.

A is incorrect because antibiotic ointment is not necessary to have in the room, and the UAP should not be instructed to handle any medications. Antibiotic ointment is not used routinely in the care of traction pin sites. The ointment will only be necessary if the pin sites become reddened or inflamed.

B is incorrect because a sequential compression device will only be used on the unaffected leg to promote circulation.

D is incorrect because a cold therapy system used for patients who have had knee surgery, not traction. This system circulates ice-cold water from a thermal container into a wrap surrounding the affected extremity to prevent swelling and provide pain relief for up to six hours.

29. The nurse is assisting a nursing student with auscultating a patient's breath sounds. Which action by the student nurse requires intervention by the nurse?

   A. Use of the bell of the stethoscope
   B. Asking the patient to sit up
   C. Placing the stethoscope on the patient's skin

179

D. Having the patient take slow, deep breaths through their mouth

Rationale:

Correct answer: A

The bell of the stethoscope is designed to listen to low-pitched sounds, such as a heart murmur. The diaphragm of the stethoscope is used to auscultate breath sounds. Normal breath sounds include bronchial sounds (heard over tracheobronchial tree) and vesicular sounds (heard over lung tissue).

B is incorrect because asking the patient to sit up is appropriate when listening to breath sounds. Sitting up facilitates easier breathing, which will allow the patient to take deeper breaths and the nurse to hear breath sounds more clearly.

C is incorrect because the stethoscope is warmed and then placed directly on the skin for auscultation.

D is incorrect because slow, deep breaths through the mouth are appropriate when auscultating breath sounds.

30. The nurse is orienting a new monitor technician for electrocardiogram (ECG) monitoring on the unit. Which of the following actions by the monitor tech requires intervention by the nurse?

    A. Uses clippers on the skin to remove hair where electrodes will be placed
    B. Tells the nurse electrodes will be changed and skin inspected every 24 hours
    C. Tells the nurse hypoallergenic electrodes are used for sensitive-skinned patients
    D. Cleanses skin with betadine before applying electrodes

Rationale:

Correct answer: D

Before applying ECG electrodes, the skin is not cleansed with betadine as some patients are sensitive or allergic to betadine. Betadine does not facilitate adherence of the electrodes to the skin. Before application of electrodes, each skin site should be cleaned thoroughly with soap and water, a non-alcohol wipe, or a 4x4 with saline to improve electrical flow. The skin should be dried vigorously to increase capillary blood flow to the tissues and ensure no moisture remains on the skin. Alcohol should not be used because it dries the skin out and may diminish electrical flow.

A is incorrect because using clippers on the skin is appropriate. Excessive hair can prevent good electrode contact.

B is incorrect because electrodes are changed and skin must be inspected every 24 hours.

C is incorrect because hypoallergenic electrodes are used for sensitive patients.

31. The medical-surgical nurse has just received the report on a patient in the ER being admitted for active tuberculosis (TB). In which of the following types of rooms, does the nurse plan to place the patient?

    A. Intensive care unit (ICU) room
    B. Private, well-ventilated room
    C. Double room because the patient will be receiving intravenous antibiotics
    D. Double room with a strict handwashing sign on the door

Rationale:

Correct answer: B

A patient admitted with active TB requires a private room with airborne precautions for isolation procedures. A negative-pressure room with several exchanges of fresh air per hour that are ventilated outside is optimal for this patient. The door must remain shut and all healthcare providers must wear PPE including a fitted N-95 respirator mask when entering the room.

A is incorrect because it is not appropriate to transfer this patient to a higher level of care.

C is incorrect because the patient must be placed in isolation regardless of antibiotics.

D is incorrect because the patient must be placed in isolation with airborne precautions.

32. The nursing student is writing a care plan for a patient scheduled for endoscopy. When the registered nurse reviews the student's care plan for the patient, which intervention does the nurse discuss with the nursing student as incorrect?

    A. Removing dentures or partial plates
    B. Removing contact lenses
    C. Allowing food and drink up to one hour before the procedure
    D. Obtaining signed consent

Rationale:

Correct answer: C

Endoscopy is a radiologic procedure in which a flexible tube with a camera is guided down the throat into the stomach. The patient must be NPO (nothing by mouth) for 6-8 hours before the procedure to prevent vomiting and aspiration. The nurse needs to discuss this with the student as incorrect.

A is incorrect because dentures or partial plates are removed before sedation is administered.

B is incorrect because contact lenses are removed before sedation is administered.

D is incorrect because informed consent must be obtained by the healthcare provider before the invasive procedure. The nursing team is not responsible for obtaining consent. (The nurse witnesses the healthcare provider explaining the procedure and answering the patient's questions, then the nurse signs as a witness.)

33. The oncology nurse is caring for a patient with ovarian cancer and believes the dose of chemotherapeutic medication prescribed by the healthcare provider is too high. When the nurse calls the healthcare provider, the office says he is out of the office for the weekend. What is the most appropriate action by the nurse?

    A. Administer the dose as ordered
    B. Call the answering service and speak with the on-call healthcare provider
    C. Hold the dose until the on-call healthcare provider makes rounds the next day
    D. Call the pharmacist and request a reduction of the dose

Rationale:

Correct answer: B

Whenever a nurse believes an order by a healthcare provider is an error, the error must be clarified with the healthcare provider or on-call provider to correct before administration of the medication at the time the error is noticed. The nurse should focus on the patient and advocate for clarification promptly.

Chemotherapy must be administered properly and as scheduled for effectiveness.

A is incorrect because any time a nurse believes an order has been written incorrectly, it is safest to contact the healthcare provider for clarification. The nurse should not administer a dose if it is believed to be written in error.

C is incorrect because missing or delaying doses of chemotherapy will decrease the effectiveness of the medication.

D is incorrect because the pharmacist cannot alter dosage until a revised order from the healthcare provider is received.

34. The new graduate nurse, observed by the nurse preceptor, is preparing to administer pyridostigmine to a patient diagnosed with myasthenia gravis. Which action by the new graduate nurse indicates safe practice when administering the medication?

    A. Have the patient take sips of water
    B. Have the patient lie down on the right side

C. Have the patient look up toward the ceiling for 30 seconds

D. Ask the patient to void prior to taking the medication

Rationale:

Correct answer: A

Myasthenia gravis is a progressive, chronic neuromuscular disease characterized by muscle weakness that descends down the body. This can affect the patient's ability to swallow effectively. Having the patient take sips of water before taking the medication helps the nurse assess ability to swallow as part of the primary assessment. Pyridostigmine is the drug of choice for MG for improvement of muscle strength. This medication should be taken at the same time every day, six hours between doses. Adverse reactions include seizures, bradycardia, and hypotension. The nurse should have atropine injection available if needed.

B is incorrect because it is an inappropriate action and places the patient at risk for aspiration. The patient should be upright when taking the medication and during meals. When administering anything PO to an MG patient, the nurse should carefully assess for swallowing difficulty and aspiration.

C is incorrect because it is an inappropriate action. Looking up towards the ceiling does not facilitate easy swallowing.

D is incorrect because there is no need to have the patient void before taking the medication.

35. The licensed practical nurse (LPN) is providing care to a patient with end-stage heart failure under the supervision of the registered nurse (RN). The patient is disinterested in care, hygiene activities, and is refusing to talk. Which statement by the LPN demonstrates the RN needs to educate the LPN on therapeutic communication?

    A. "You seem very quiet today."
    B. "What are you feeling right now?"
    C. "Why don't you want to get up?"
    D. "Tell me about your difficulty with sleep."

Rationale:

Correct answer: C

End-stage heart failure is the end of the disease process of heart failure, and many patients experience depression, sadness, and grief, among many other emotions. Patients may not know why they don't want to do a certain activity or why they feel a certain way, so a *why* question is inappropriate. Asking "why?" is non-therapeutic and can make the patient feel they need to defend themselves.

A is incorrect because it is acknowledging the patient's behavior and is an appropriate statement. This is reflective of the patient's mood and can encourage a healthy nurse-client relationship.

B is incorrect because it encourages the patient to identify feelings and is an appropriate response. A component of therapeutic communication is to focus on the here-and-now.

D is incorrect because it encourages the patient to explore reasons behind the sleep difficulties and is an appropriate response.

36. The unlicensed assistive personnel (UAP) is caring for a patient with a nasogastric tube (NGT) that was placed following gastric surgery the previous day under the observation of the registered nurse. Which action by the UAP requires intervention by the nurse?

    A. Hands the patient a cup of ice water
    B. Performs oral care for the patient
    C. Hands the patient an oral swab
    D. Pins the NGT to the patient's gown

Rationale:

Correct answer: A

Following gastric surgery, the patient will be NPO (nothing by mouth) in order for the stomach to rest. The patient will remain NPO until bowel sounds have returned, the NGT is removed, and the patient can swallow effectively. The nurse should intervene if the UAP hands the patient a cup of ice water as this will lead to possible nausea and vomiting, even with the NGT in place.

B is incorrect because oral care is important for the patient who has an NGT in place. Oral care can help decrease the risk for infection and provides comfort as the mucus membranes of the mouth can become dry and uncomfortable when the patient is NPO.

C is incorrect because the patient can participate in their own oral care with an NGT in place.

D is incorrect because pinning the NGT to the patient's gown can prevent pulling on the patient's nares and forming of a pressure ulcer.

37. The nurse manager has implemented an update in the process by which nursing staff is to document nursing care in the patient records. One nurse is resistant to the update and refuses to facilitate the change process. Which approach is most appropriate for the nurse manager to use with the resistant nurse?

A. Ignore the behavior

B. Tell the nurse to work somewhere else

C. Confront the nurse and ask about their feelings regarding the update

D. Tell the nurse to comply with the update

Rationale:

Correct answer: C

When resistance to change is met, confrontation can benefit both parties. Allowing the nurse to verbalize their feelings and opinions related to the change can help solve the problem. An open discussion about the resistance to change will allow the nurse manager to assess the reasons for the resistance and identify any barriers to learning the new documentation system. Then the nurse manager can assist the staff nurse in making the necessary changes to adapt to the new process.

A is incorrect because ignoring the behavior does not address the problem.

B is incorrect because telling the nurse to leave does not address the problem.

D is incorrect because telling the nurse to comply does not guarantee that they will. They have already shown resistance and refusal, so this does not address the problem.

38. The new nurse manager of the cardiac unit wants to schedule a strategic planning workshop with the staff to assist with effective and efficient unit management. Which of the following activities is not a characteristic of this workshop?

    A. Determining direction of the unit

    B. Focusing on daily tasks

    C. Long-term goal setting

    D. Focusing on success of the unit

Rationale:

Correct answer: B

A nursing strategic plan creates a shared vision, reinforces understanding the current state of nursing services, and helps to identify strengths and gaps within the unit's nursing department. Goals and actions for achieving those goals are outlined in the strategic plan. Strategic planning for a new nurse manager of a unit does not focus on daily tasks; this is attributed to operational planning.

A is incorrect because strategic planning includes determining direction of the unit.

C is incorrect because strategic planning includes long-term goal setting.

D is incorrect because strategic planning includes focusing on success.

39. The nurse manager is interested in improving staff input and leadership on the medical-surgical unit as seen in magnet hospitals. Which of the following choices describes the style of leadership the nurse manager is looking for?

   A. Leadership behavior determined by the relationship between personalities and specific situations
   B. Leadership shared at the point of care
   C. Heavy reliance on vision and inspiring members for achievement of results
   D. Belief that people are good and do not need close supervision

Rationale:

Correct answer: B

Shared governance is the style of leadership often seen in magnet hospitals and leads to improved patient outcomes, more staff involvement, and increased nurse retention.

A is incorrect because it describes situational leadership. A situational leader is flexible and adaptive to the existing work environment and the needs of the organization. The management approach is modified between leadership styles to suit the requirements of the organization.

C is incorrect because it describes democratic leadership. This type of leader encourages open communication and staff participation in decisions. Staff are given responsibility and accountability and receive feedback regarding their performance. A democratic nursing leader values relationships and focuses on quality improvement of systems and processes, rather than on mistakes of individual team members.

D is incorrect because it describes laissez-faire leadership. This style is the least

effective in promoting purposeful interaction between the leader and employees for organizational success

40. A new patient care manager is updating knowledge of theories of management and leadership for role effectiveness. It is learned that one type of management is characterized by low concern for service and high concern for staff. Which management style is this?

   A. Organization man
   B. Impoverished management
   C. Country club management
   D. Team management

Rationale:

Correct answer: C

The country club management style is characterized by low concern for delivery of services and concern for staff as the number one priority. The primary goal is to create a comfortable work atmosphere in which all staff, including the manager, are content, leading to a comfortable experience for clients.

A is incorrect because, in organization man, the manager is concerned about the organization as a whole. This is also known as a "middle of the road" leadership approach, achieving adequate performance along with satisfactory employee morale. These leaders tend to avoid conflict and not push employees too hard with hopes of adequate job performance.

B is incorrect because, in impoverished management, low concern for people and tasks is exhibited. These leaders exhibit low concern for both the results of tasks and for interpersonal relationships and may give the impression that they only perform to sustain employment.

D is incorrect because team management has high concern for both people and tasks. These leaders create strongly structured tasks, set clear goals, and track progress. Active participation and teamwork are promoted and individuals are empowered to keep them motivated.

41. The nurse manager of the telemetry unit is interested in promoting a positive organizational culture in the unit. Which of the following behaviors by the staff indicate this has been achieved?

    A. Obedience and no complaining
    B. Competitive and perfectionist
    C. Powerful and oppositional
    D. Proactive and caring of each other

Rationale:

Correct answer: D

A positive organizational culture on a unit is characterized by proactive behaviors and demonstration of care for all the members of the team. A positive nursing culture reduces patient mortality and nurse emotional exhaustion and improves nurses' health, job satisfaction, retention, organizational commitment, and intent to stay in their position.

A is incorrect because obedience and no complaints are characteristic of an authoritarian or autocratic leadership nursing style.

B is incorrect because competition and perfectionism are not components of a positive organizational culture. When nurses display competition between peers, both staff job satisfaction and patient outcomes can be negatively affected.

C is incorrect because power and opposition are characteristics of a defiant staff.

42. The staff educator nurse is orienting a new nurse about channel and lines of communication. Which of the following resources provides information about communication in the organization?

   A. Procedure manual
   B. Organizational structure
   C. Policy handbook
   D. Job description

Rationale:

Correct answer: B

The channels of communication and authority are included in the organizational structure. This will let staff members know who directly reports to whom and specifies different levels of authority.

A is incorrect because the procedure manual does not give any information about communication or chain of command. The procedure manual will give detailed instructions for specific procedures such as blood administration, administering nebulizer therapy, or maintenance of an intravenous line.

C is incorrect because the policy handbook includes policies related to patient care and organizational safety, not specifically communication. The policy handbook will contain information related to patient rights, cultural diversity, core measures, medication error reporting, etc.

D is incorrect because the job description delineates responsibilities of a specific job role, not communication. An example of a hospital RN job description is, "promotes and restores patients' health by utilizing the nursing process, collaborating with healthcare providers and multi-disciplinary team-members, and providing physical and psychological support to patients and families."

43. The nurse manager is interested in transformational leadership on the cardiovascular unit. Which of the following is characteristic of transformational leadership?

   A. Vision is used as essence of leadership
   B. Full trust and confidence are maintained in direct reports
   C. Possesses innate charisma for leadership that makes others feel good in their presence
   D. Is a servant to the followers rather than the followers serving the leader

Rationale:

Correct answer: A

Transformational leadership is characterized by vision as the core of the leadership style. The transformational nurse leader recognizes areas in which change is needed and guides change by inspiring followers and creating a sense of commitment.

B is incorrect because full trust and confidence in direct reports are not characteristic of transformational leadership.

C is incorrect because these are qualities of a charismatic leader.

D is incorrect because this is characteristic of servant leadership.

44. The new nurse is learning about the nursing process and nursing leadership at the bedside. Which of the following options follows the nursing process framework while planning, organizing, and directing patient care?

    A. Coordinating with the multidisciplinary team members
    B. Consulting with the healthcare provider
    C. Collaborative effort with the patient in preparing nursing care plans
    D. Involving the patient's family members in care

Rationale:

Correct answer: C

The priority needs of the patient are best expressed by the patient, so collaborating with the patient when preparing nursing care plans is most effective. This is the answer choice that is the most patient-focused.

A is incorrect because multidisciplinary team members are not vital to the steps of the nursing process. Certainly, other disciplines are essential components of providing good care overall, but the nursing process is five steps that are nurse-patient focused.

B is incorrect because consulting with the healthcare provider is not necessarily a component of any of the five steps of the nursing process.

D is incorrect because it may be important to involve patient relatives but does not best meet the patient's needs.

45. The new charge nurse is learning about staffing effectiveness. The charge nurse knows there must be adequate staff for accomplishing certain purposes, including all of the following except:

A. Covering all shifts adequately

B. Meeting the needs of all patients

C. Allowing time for professional growth and development of staff

D. Floating staff to other departments as needed

Rationale:

Correct answer: D

Floating staff to meet needs in other units is not the purpose of staffing effectiveness. This is performed by a nursing supervisor in a centralized, higher-level model.

A is incorrect because covering all shifts adequately is a component of staffing effectiveness. Other components include preparedness for new admissions, partnering new graduate nurses with adequately trained preceptors, and maintaining the nurse-patient ratio for the unit.

B is incorrect because meeting needs of patients is a component of staffing effectiveness.

C is incorrect because professional growth and development time is a component of staffing effectiveness. Staff nurses must consistently be allowed time to review policies, learn about new changes being implemented, and train for new procedures and practices.

46. The new nurse manager of the cardiac unit learns that patient satisfaction has decreased to 65% and staff morale is low. The nurse manager would like to plan and initiate changes to turn things around on the unit. Which of the following is a priority action for the nurse manager?

A. Schedule a staff meeting and include this on the agenda

B. Develop an action plan on how to correct the problems

C. Seek assistance from the director

D. Observe the operations of the unit for two more weeks to determine underlying causes

Rationale:

Correct answer: A

Discussion of the issues during a staff meeting will encourage participation of the staff in resolving the problems. This will increase compliance of the staff in any changes that are made.

B is incorrect because an action plan cannot be adequately developed without assessing the situation and obtaining input from the staff, first.

C is incorrect because the new nurse manager should first take steps to get more information about the situation and involve the staff before going up the vertical chain of command.

D is incorrect because this delays addressing the problems. Holding a staff meeting with the experienced nurses on the unit will give the manager the most pertinent information the most quickly, in order to set goals and begin planning for changes.

47. The nurse manager has noted increasing frustration of staff due to fatigue and short staffing. Which action by the nurse manager takes priority?

    A. Develop a plan to address short staffing and implement it

    B. Identify internal and external causes

    C. Evaluate overall impact of frustration

    D. Schedule a staff meeting for group interaction

Rationale:

Correct answer: A

Staff can contribute to problem-solving related to many issues, but when short staffing is the issue, the nurse manager doesn't need to collaborate with the staff. Energy should be focused on hiring new nurses. Other options include obtaining float staff, temporary nurses, agency nurses, or additional unlicensed assistive personnel to help fix the staffing issue.

B is incorrect because the nurse manager already knows the cause of the frustration: fatigue and short staffing. No more information is needed at this time about causes; the manager should address the problem by implementing a plan to either hire more nurses or close beds on the unit until the staffing issue has been resolved.

C is incorrect because it is more important to address the staffing issue than to evaluate the effects of the problem. Short staffing can have a negative effect on patient safety, so the number one priority is to fix the staffing problem.

D is incorrect because the staff is already fatigued from short staffing. Scheduling a staff meeting at this time will only contribute to the fatigue. Input from the staff isn't needed in this situation. The nurse manager should focus time and efforts on a solution to get the unit back to safe staffing levels. This will have the best outcome for both patients and nursing team members.

48. The cardiac unit nurse supervisor is aware of a nurse experiencing burnout. Which of the following actions by the nurse supervisor is best?

    A. Ignore the observations as it will resolve itself

    B. Offer assistance and allow the nurse to express feelings

    C. Transfer the nurse to a less acute unit

D. Remind the nurse of the importance of loyalty to the organization

Rationale:

Correct answer: B

Offering physical assistance with workload is important for patient safety. Reaching out to the nurse and allowing self-expression will help identify the problem. Nurse burnout can have three components: emotional exhaustion, depersonalization, and dissatisfaction with personal achievements. The nurse supervisor can offer the following suggestions to help alleviate burnout: plan your day at the beginning of the shift and prioritize efficiently, say *no* to new assignments if you feel you can't perform them safely, delegate appropriately to assistive personnel, and seek help from the charge nurse when you're getting behind.

A is incorrect because it is inappropriate and non-therapeutic to ignore nurse burnout. Burnout, if unaddressed, can impact the safety and quality of patient care.

C is incorrect because transferring the nurse does not address the burnout. This action makes the assumption that patient acuity level is the cause of the burnout.

D is incorrect because reminding the nurse of loyalty to the organization does not address the problem of burnout. This is dismissive and does not show concern for the nurse or patient safety.

49. The quality control officer is developing a plan to meet goals and objectives of the nursing department. Which task should the quality control officer complete first?

  A. Identify nursing department values
  B. Identify strengths and weaknesses of the organization
  C. Measure actual performance
  D. Identify structure, process, outcome standards, and criteria

Rationale:

Correct answer: A

Identifying values will set the guiding principles for operations of the organization.

B is incorrect because identifying strengths and weaknesses is a component of quality improvement, not goal and objective planning.

C is incorrect because measuring actual performance will be done after the values have been identified.

D is incorrect because although identifying structure, process, outcome standards, and criteria is important, it is not done first.

50. The Chief Nursing Operator (CNO) is working on designing an organizational structure that utilizes open communication that flows in all directions and involves the facility staff in making decisions. Which of the following forms of organizational structure is this?

    A. Matrix
    B. Informal
    C. Decentralized
    D. Centralized

Rationale:

Correct answer: C

A decentralized organizational structure allows for open communication that flows in all directions as well as involving staff in the decision-making process.

A is incorrect because matrix structure divides authority by function and by project (staff report to two supervisors). Matrix structure is uncommonly used in nursing.

B is incorrect because informal structure develops around social or project groups and is based on camaraderie. An informal structure may be found among staff nurses but would not likely include staff nurses and the CNO.

D is incorrect because centralized structure does not involve staff in decision-making.

51. The nurse manager of the medical-surgical unit is preparing nursing process standards for the unit. Which of the following is *not* an example of a process standard?

    A. Patient education will be provided for all patients and family members
    B. Consent will be obtained before all procedures
    C. Patients will report 96% satisfaction rate before discharge
    D. Initial assessment will be completed within 24 hours of admission

Rationale:

Correct answer: C

Process standards are specific to operations of the unit. Nursing process standards describe competent level of care required in each of the five phases of the nursing process. They reflect a desired and achievable level of performance against which a nurse's actual performance can be compared.

The main purpose of nursing process standards is to direct and maintain safe and clinically competent nursing practice. Patient satisfaction is not directly reflected by nursing process standards, but rather, is an outcome resulting from patient care.

A is incorrect because patient education is a process standard. Every step of the nursing process involves educating the patient (about what the nurse has assessed, what it means to the nurse, intervention plans for achieving good outcomes, and the method of evaluating those outcomes.)

B is incorrect because obtaining consent is a process standard. The nurse obtains consent for all nursing procedures and also ensures that signed consent is obtained for any invasive procedure to be performed by the healthcare provider.

D is incorrect because initial assessment completion is a process standard.

52. The nurse manager of the medical-surgical unit is informing the nursing staff of nursing procedures to be followed. What type of standards is the nurse manager referring to?

   A. Criteria
   B. Process
   C. Outcome
   D. Structure

Rationale:

Correct answer: B

The standards the nurse manager is referring to are process standards, which include care plans and nursing procedures to address patient needs.

A is incorrect because criteria are not a type of standard.

C is incorrect because outcome standards are not limited strictly to nursing procedures. Hospital outcomes standards include, for example, quality of transition when admitted, improvement in health-related quality of life and functional status, palliative care symptom control, surgical outcomes, and efficiency.

D is incorrect because structure is not a type of standard.

53. The nurse manager of the surgical unit is talking with the nurses about criteria. Which of the following are characteristic of criteria?

   A. A method chosen to achieve a goal
   B. Step-by-step guidelines

C. Level of nursing care that is agreed upon

D. Used to measure level of nursing care

Rationale:

Correct answer: D

The standard of care is measured by specific characteristics, or criteria. Each of the criteria is a specific, measurable item that reflects expected end results of the nursing process.

A is incorrect because a method or plan chosen to bring about a desired future, such as achievement of a goal or solution to a problem, is a strategy, not criteria.

B is incorrect because criteria are not step-by-step guidelines.

C is incorrect because criteria are not used for agreeing on level of nursing care.

54. The nursing director is working with the new nurse manager to ensure tasks are carried out as planned. Which of the following are not included in the controlling process?

 A. Reviewing policies of the facility
 B. Instructing the professional practice committee to prepare facility policies
 C. Checking if activities work with the schedule
 D. Evaluating credentials of all healthcare staff members

Rationale:

Correct answer: B

A is incorrect because policy review is an important component of the controlling process.

C is incorrect because checking to be sure that assigned tasks and activities fit into the staff nurses' daily work schedule is included in the controlling process.

D is incorrect because evaluating staff credentials is an important legal and safety measure included in the controlling process.

55. The charge nurse is completing informal appraisals of the staff during daily rounds. Which is not a benefit of informal appraisals?

 A. Staff are observed in their natural work setting
 B. Evaluation can provide information for a formal evaluation
 C. Incidental confrontation and collaboration is allowed
 D. Evaluation is based on subjective data collected systematically

Rationale:

Correct answer: D

Collecting subjective data systematically is not achieved with an informal appraisal. When performing an informal appraisal, the charge nurse objectively observes the staff nurse performing in the natural work environment. The charge nurse should avoid making presumptions or using personal opinions when observing the staff nurse. Objective data to be collected includes timeliness of patient assessment, precision of documentation, accurate medication administration, and ability to adhere to the daily work schedule and manage patient workload.

A is incorrect because staff observation in the natural work setting is a benefit of informal appraisals.

B is incorrect because informal appraisals can provide information for a formal evaluation to be completed at a later time.

C is incorrect because incidental confrontation and collaboration are a benefit of informal appraisals. If the charge nurse notices the staff nurse performing a procedure inappropriately, for example, the charge nurse can discuss the issue with the staff nurse right there at the bedside and offer support and teaching to correct the error.

56. The new nurse manager knows that performance appraisals consist of all of the following except:
    A. Using agency standards to guide the appraisal
    B. Determining areas of strength and weakness
    C. Focusing activity on correction of identified behavior
    D. Setting specific activities for individual performance

Rationale:

Correct answer: C

A performance appraisal is designed to reflect positive and negative aspects of performance, not to correct behavior.

A is incorrect because agency standards are used to guide the performance appraisal process.

B is incorrect because the purpose of a performance appraisal is to determine strengths and weaknesses.

D is incorrect because specific activities must be set before the performance appraisal can take place. Activities to be evaluated may include starting an IV, drawing blood from a central line, safely transferring a patient to the ICU, discharge teaching, and proper documentation of nursing care.

57. One of the nurses approaches the nurse manager on the medical-surgical unit with a problem. The nurse manager tells the nurse to come to the office at the end of their shift to discuss the concern. Which conflict resolution strategy did the nurse manager use?

    A. Compromise
    B. Smoothing
    C. Avoidance
    D. Restriction

Rationale:

Correct answer: C

Avoidance is an unassertive approach to conflict. Managers who avoid neither pursue their own needs, goals, or concerns immediately nor assist others to pursue theirs. This mode could cause conflict to be postponed or to escalate. The nurse manager has avoided talking about the problem in the current situation and has postponed it. The problem remains unsolved.

This is a potentially dangerous conflict resolution strategy because, in the meantime, patient care could be compromised and patient safety is at risk. The nurse manager should address the concern at the time it is brought to attention, or shortly thereafter. The nurse manager is legally and ethically required to address problems as they arise and not delay safe patient care.

A is incorrect because compromise is when both parties come to a resolution together. Compromise requires assertiveness and cooperation on the part of everyone involved and requires maturity and confidence. Compromise often involves negotiation, which is a learned skill that is developed over time. This approach to conflict resolution often results in each individual's ability to meet their most important priorities as much of the time as possible.

B is incorrect because smoothing is not a conflict resolution strategy.

D is incorrect because restriction is not a conflict resolution strategy.

58. The new nurse manager is learning about conflict. Which of the following is not true regarding conflict?

    A. Conflict can be destructive
    B. Conflict can result in decreased level of performance
    C. Conflict can create leaders
    D. Conflict is detrimental and should be prevented

Rationale:

Correct answer: D

Conflicts can be beneficial because they identify issues that can be solved. Team members can be more conscientious of their work when they know they are being observed.

A is incorrect because conflict can be destructive. Some results of inappropriate conflict resolution include negativity, resistance, increased frustration, division of groups, weakened relationships, and decreased productivity.

B is incorrect because conflict can result in decreased level of performance.

C is incorrect because conflict does not always have a negative outcome. Constructive conflict resolution can lead to individual growth as people work together to solve problems. Groups may become more unified as a result of positive conflict resolution, thus increasing commitment, satisfaction, productivity, and ultimately identifying potential future nurse leaders.

59. The nurse manager of the oncology unit is interested in implementing primary nursing to deliver patient care on the unit. Which of the following does not characterize primary nursing?

  A. The primary nurse performs a comprehensive initial assessment
  B. The primary nurse provides care for 4-to-5 patients while admitted
  C. The primary nurse provides care with a team of nurses to a group of patients
  D. The primary nurse delegates to the LPN for a group of patients

Rationale:

Correct answer: C

This statement describes team nursing. Primary nursing is a system of nursing care that focuses on continuity of care by assigning one RN responsible for a group of patients throughout their stay in a hospital unit. This primary nurse administers some and coordinates all aspects of the patient's nursing care throughout the patient's length of stay. Primary nursing emphasizes the therapeutic nurse-client relationship.

A is incorrect because a characteristic of primary nursing is that the primary nurse completes the initial assessment and coordinates all other nursing care for the patient, even when not on shift.

B is incorrect because, with primary nursing care, the RN assumes responsibility for a group of patients. The RN is often teamed with an LPN/LVN and/or unlicensed assistive personnel (UAP) who together provide complete patient care.

D is incorrect because proper delegation is a key component of primary nursing. When RNs supervise LPNs and UAPs in providing patient care, benefits include lowered labor costs, well-coordinated care, and increased patient satisfaction and safety.

60. The telemetry nurse educator is orienting a new group of nurses to the telemetry unit. The new nurses are learning about required *floating* to other units when census is high. The nurse educator tells the new nurses if they are assigned to *float* to a unit they are unfamiliar with, their role is to:

    A. Refuse the assignment
    B. Notify the telemetry nurse educator
    C. Report to the new unit for brief orientation and safe task identification
    D. Contact the nursing supervisor and request to float to a different unit

Rationale:

Correct answer: C

Floating is frequently used in facilities when census is high, and staffing is inadequate on a particular unit. Nurses' skills are transferable, and the RN can safely work in a unit where familiar tasks are identified The RN is competent to perform general assessment and care for most hospitalized patients. The float nurse should report to the assigned unit for a brief orientation and identify what types of tasks and procedures they are competent in performing. Floating is generally not required in highly specialized areas, such as ICU, oncology, and ER. Nurses who care for adult patients are rarely expected to float to a pediatrics unit.

A is incorrect because the RN's skills are transferable and refusal does not focus on the patient. The RN can request stable patients and utilize the assistance of the charge nurse when floating to a different unit.

B is incorrect because the telemetry nurse educator is not responsible for floating practices. If needed, the nurse educator on the new floor can assist the float nurse.

D is incorrect because the nursing supervisor makes the unit assignments for floating and this decision should not be challenged by the RN.

61. The nurse is working with a new unlicensed assistive personnel (UAP) caring for a group of patients. The nurse needs to intervene when the UAP performs which action?

    A. Patient returned from CABG procedure this morning; UAP assists the patient to a chair.
    B. Patient with COPD; UAP documents vital signs: BP 122/68, HR 88 bmp, RR 16/min, SpO_2 93%
    C. Patient has internal radiation in place for cervical cancer; UAP empties the patient's urinal in the toilet.
    D. Patient is recovering from cerebrovascular accident five days ago; UAP ambulates patient in the hallway.

Rationale:

Correct answer: A

This is an inappropriate action by the UAP because the first time the patient is assisted to the chair, the RN should assist and assess for complications during the transfer. UAP can assist with transfer for stable patients, but the first transfer post-op requires the RN.

B is incorrect because documenting vital signs is an appropriate action by the UAP. These are expected VS for a patient with COPD, so the UAP does not need to notify the primary RN. Any time the UAP collects abnormal VS, the data should be reported to the primary RN immediately.

C is incorrect because emptying a urinal in the toilet is an appropriate action by the UAP. Output must be recorded in the patient record. With internal radiation in place, the urine can be safely flushed, as it does not contain any radioactive material.

D is incorrect because the UAP can ambulate a stable patient. This patient experienced a CVA five days ago, and no information suggests any complications.

62. The nurse manager overhears one of the staff nurses complaining about the manager's style of leadership. Which of the following actions would be appropriate by the nurse manager?

 A. Confront the nurse and suggest the critical comments stop
 B. Propose solutions to the negative comments
 C. Encourage the nurse to discuss the negative comments with the nurse manager
 D. Encourage the nurse to maintain a positive attitude for the general benefit of the nursing team morale and patient care

Rationale:

Correct answer: C

Encouraging the nurse to discuss negative comments will help identify the problems and concerns in a democratic manner. This will help the nurse and manager discuss potential solutions together.

A is incorrect because confrontation does not help identify the problem and this is dismissive. It is more important for the manager to address the nurse's concerns and identify goals for resolution.

B is incorrect because solutions cannot be proposed based on comments overheard. The nurse should be encouraged to share concerns openly in one-on-one discussion with the manager before solutions can be generated.

D is incorrect because this does not allow the nurse to share concerns or identify the problem. The nurse manager should not dismiss concerns of the staff.

63. The registered nurse is working with a nursing student who is preparing a patient for renal angiography. Which action by the nursing student would necessitate intervention by the registered nurse?

    A. Checking the patient's renal function lab results
    B. Verified allergies
    C. Checked for signed consent for the procedure
    D. Checked for signed general anesthesia consent for the procedure

Rationale:

Correct answer: D

Consent for the procedure is performed under local anesthesia to examine the vasculature of the renal system. General anesthesia is not used for this procedure.

A is incorrect because checking renal function lab results is an appropriate action by the student. Contrast dye is metabolized by the kidneys, so checking for baseline renal function is a safety measure before the procedure. If kidney function is already impaired prior to the study, less dye may be used, and the patient will be monitored more closely during the angiography.

B is incorrect because verifying allergies before a procedure that uses contrast medium is appropriate. If the patient has an allergy to iodine or shellfish, the RN must notify the healthcare provider and anticipate a different diagnostic procedure (without contrast medium) will be used.

C is incorrect because a signed consent is necessary for any invasive procedure.

64. The nurse manager of the telemetry unit has learned that two staff nurses have been experiencing a conflict with each other and it is affecting the work environment negatively. Which action by the nurse manager is most appropriate?

    A. Offer temporary workload relief and encourage the nurses to work it out in the break room
    B. Confront the nurses and tell them to stop the behavior towards each other
    C. Meet with the nurses and facilitate a discussion to identify the problem
    D. Notify human resources of the conflict

Rationale:

Correct answer: C

Conflict between nurses can have a negative effect on the work environment and affects patient care and outcomes. The nurse manager should meet with the nurses experiencing the conflict to facilitate a discussion about working out the conflict.

A is incorrect because the two nurses involved in the conflict should resolve the conflict with the help of the charge nurse or manager. A mediator is helpful in maintaining neutrality and proposing resolution.

B is incorrect because confrontation can lead to an argument and will not fix the issue. This does not address the underlying problem.

D is incorrect because the manager should attempt to identify the problem before involving human resources.

65. The registered nurse (RN) has delegated subcutaneous medication administration to the licensed practical nurse (LPN). Which of the following statements describes delegation most accurately?

    A. Subcutaneous medication administration must be taught to the LPN by the RN
    B. The responsibility for medication administration is with the LPN
    C. The RN must observe the LPN perform medication administration
    D. The RN is accountable for quality patient care delivery

Rationale:

Correct answer: D

The RN is in a position to delegate certain aspects of patient care, but the RN is ultimately responsible for the patient and the tasks performed. Steps for appropriate delegation include define the task, specify which patient should receive the delegated task, match the task to an individual who possesses the skill and ability to safely complete the task, provide communication about expected outcome of the task, and answer questions. The RN should not delegate: total control, discipline issues, highly technical tasks, or during a crisis.

A is incorrect because it is inappropriate to delegate a task the LPN is unfamiliar with. If the LPN requires teaching about administration of subcutaneous medication injection, that is the responsibility of the nurse manager. The RN should give the injection.

B is incorrect because the RN is ultimately responsible for medication administration.

C is incorrect because the RN does not have to observe an LPN performing tasks delegated by the RN. The RN should clarify whether written or verbal documentation is required after the task is completed.

66. The nursing director is reviewing staffing patterns on the medical-surgical units. The nurse director knows which of the following is an advantage of decentralized staffing?

A. Increased control over activities

B. Time conservation

C. Compatible with the computer system

D. Promotes interpersonal relationships

Rationale:

Correct answer: D

Staffing may be centralized or decentralized. With centralized staffing, one department is responsible for staffing all units, including float staff, on-call staff, and those who call off. With decentralized staffing, charge nurses or managers use multiple factors (including staff nurse input) to determine the staffing level required for the shift. Decentralized staffing promotes interpersonal relationships by allowing staff members to make decisions and solve problems within the team. This model of staffing provides many opportunities for interaction among members of the nursing team, promoting interpersonal relationships.

A is incorrect because decentralized staffing transfers much of the control from top management to the management of the nursing units. Staff nurses are allowed to give input and creativity when planning nursing staffing and care. This is less controlling than centralized staffing.

B is incorrect because decentralized staffing has no relation to time management.

C is incorrect because decentralized staffing has no effect on computer systems.

67. The new emergency room nurse is preparing to draw a blood alcohol level on a patient. The experienced emergency room nurse should intervene if the new nurse chooses which item?

A. Tourniquet
B. Alcohol swab
C. Blood tube
D. Vacutainer with needle

Rationale:

Correct answer: B

Isopropyl alcohol swabs or any solution with alcohol cannot be used as skin prep when drawing blood for a blood alcohol level. This could falsely elevate the serum level and invalidate the test. The experienced emergency room nurse should intervene and suggest betadine swabs. (If the patient is allergic to betadine, another skin prep solution that does not contain alcohol should be used.)

A is incorrect because a tourniquet is appropriate for blood draw. The tourniquet is placed 4-10 inches above the needle insertion site. When the tourniquet is applied, venous blood flow returning to the heart is slowed. The veins below the level of the tourniquet are distended, becoming more pronounced and easier to see and feel.

C is incorrect because a blood tube is necessary for collection of the sample and transfer to the lab for analysis.

D is incorrect because a vacutainer with needle is necessary.

68. The nurse is performing sterile wound irrigation in the emergency room. When the unlicensed assistive personnel (UAP) enters the room to inform the nurse the healthcare provider is on the phone asking to speak to the nurse, which action is appropriate by the nurse?

    A.   Have the healthcare provider on the phone wait while finishing the wound irrigation

    B.   Cover the wound and answer the phone

    C.   Have the UAP get a phone number so the nurse can call the healthcare provider once the wound irrigation is complete

    D.   Ask the UAP to complete the procedure so the nurse can take the phone call

Rationale:

Correct answer: C

Wound irrigation should be completed by the nurse due to risk of infection and because it is a sterile procedure. It is most appropriate to call the healthcare provider back once the procedure is completed.

A is incorrect because requesting the healthcare provider wait on the phone may delay care of other patients.

B is incorrect because, due to the risk of infection, the sterile procedure should be completed in one sitting, at the bedside. It is inappropriate to stop a sterile procedure halfway through to take a phone call.

D is incorrect because it is not within the UAP scope of practice to perform sterile wound irrigation.

69. The community health nurse is interested in providing primary prevention for a community at risk for hypertension. Which of the following interventions by the community health nurse is a primary intervention?

    A.   Encouraging attendance at hypertension screening events

    B.   Encouraging regular visits with the healthcare provider

    C.   Providing education on decreasing salt use

D.   Offering a community support group for chronic hypertension patients

Rationale:

Correct answer: C

A primary prevention is an intervention that prevents illness, injury, and potential problems from occurring. Provision of education regarding decreased salt use in the diet is a primary prevention. Primary prevention involves preventing exposure to hazards that cause disease or injury, modifying unhealthy lifestyle factors that can lead to disease or injury, and increasing resistance to disease or injury should exposure occur. Other examples of primary prevention for hypertension include education about low-fat diet, active lifestyle, and avoiding smoking.

A is incorrect because a screening event is a secondary prevention. Secondary hypertension prevention aims to reduce the impact of hypertension. This is done by screening and detecting hypertension in its earliest stages and implementing exercise programs to reduce blood pressure.

B is incorrect because healthcare provider visits are a secondary prevention.

D is incorrect because this is an example of tertiary prevention: helping people manage long-term health problems in order to maximize their level of functionality and improve quality of life and life expectancy.

70.   The nurse is orienting a new LPN/LVN on the medical unit caring for a patient with chlamydia. When the nurse delegates urinary catheter insertion to the LPN/LVN for this patient, which personal protective equipment (PPE) does the nurse advise the LPN/LVN to don?

   A.   Gloves and mask
   B.   Gloves and gown
   C.   Gown and mask
   D.   Gloves

Rationale:

Correct answer: D

The nurse should advise the LPN/LVN to don gloves for urinary catheter insertion in the patient with chlamydia because standard precautions are sufficient for protection against this sexually transmitted infection. Chlamydia is transmitted via mucous membrane contact and the incubation period is 1-3 weeks. This STI may cause sterility, and patients infected with chlamydia are required to notify all sexual contacts about the infection.

A is incorrect because a mask is unnecessary for protection against chlamydia.

B is incorrect because a gown is unnecessary for protection against chlamydia.

C is incorrect because a gown and mask are unnecessary for protection against chlamydia.

71. The nurse is observing an unlicensed assistive personnel (UAP) caring for a patient admitted for cystitis that has an indwelling urinary catheter. The nurse provides the UAP with instructions for urinary catheter care and makes sure the UAP understands to:

   A. Loop the drainage bag tubing under the leg
   B. Replace the catheter with a new one if urine flow is obstructed
   C. Use soap and water for cleansing the perineal area
   D. Hang the drainage bag at the bladder level

Rationale:

Correct answer: C

In order to prevent infection or prolonged infection with cystitis, proper care of the urinary catheter is performed with mild soap and water to the perineal area twice a day and after bowel movements.

A is incorrect because looping the drainage bag tubing does not promote drainage.

B is incorrect because it is not within the UAP's scope of practice to replace the urinary catheter. If obstruction is noted, the UAP should notify the RN. Inserting a new urinary catheter increases risk for infection. The RN will first assess the system and determine if repositioning the tubing facilitates drainage, eliminating the need for new catheter insertion.

D is incorrect because the drainage bag should be kept below the level of the bladder to prevent reflux of urine and maintain drainage flow.

72. The experienced ER nurse is orienting a new ER nurse when a patient is brought to the hospital with multiple gunshot wounds. Which of the following actions by the new nurse would necessitate intervention by the experienced nurse?

   A. Initiates a chain of custody log
   B. Gives the family the patient's wallet and clothing
   C. Cuts the clothing along seams and avoids cutting bullet holes
   D. Places the patient's belongings in a labeled, sealed paper bag

Rationale:

Correct answer: B

The new ER nurse should never give potential evidence to a patient's family. Potential evidence must be handled extremely carefully by hospital staff until it can be turned over to law enforcement authorities. Rules for handling evidence include limiting access to the belongings and evidence, initiating a log of custody for movement of evidence, and carefully removing clothing.

A is incorrect because a chain of custody log is necessary.

C is incorrect because careful cutting of clothing is necessary to preserve evidence.

D is incorrect because placing patient belongings in a labeled, sealed paper bag is necessary.

73. The nurse is orienting a new unlicensed assistive personnel (UAP) to the oncology floor. While observing the UAP perform handwashing, which action by the UAP requires intervention by the nurse?

    A. Keeps hands lower than the elbows
    B. Dries from forearm to fingers
    C. Washes hands continuously for 15 seconds
    D. Uses 3 mL of soap

Rationale:

Correct answer: B

The nurse should intervene if the UAP dries from forearm down to fingers after handwashing. Drying should be done from the fingers up to the forearms then the paper towel is used to turn off the faucet and discarded.

A is incorrect because the hands should be kept lower than the elbows during handwashing.

C is incorrect because hands should be washed vigorously for 15-20 seconds, covering all surfaces of the hands and fingers. (Hot water should be avoided because it can dry the skin.)

D is incorrect because 3 to 5 mL of soap should be used.

74. The new intensive care unit (ICU) nurse is preparing to apply a cooling pad for a patient after cardiac arrest. The charge nurse intervenes when the new nurse does which of the following?

    A. Checks the patient's temperature every four hours
    B. Places the cooling pad on the bed and covers it with a sheet
    C. Keeps the patient dry while using the cooling pad
    D. Checks the patient's skin condition before, during, and after use of the cooling pad

Rationale:

Correct answer: A

Cardiac arrest decreases O_2 and blood to the brain, which can lead to cerebral edema. The nurse is initiating hypothermia protocol, which is used for 24 hours after cardiac arrest to cool the body. The cooling blanket is used underneath the patient to decrease the patient's body temperature to 92°F to 94°F (33.3°C to 34.4°C), which must be monitored closely with a urinary catheter with temperature probe or rectal probe for hourly monitoring. Hypothermia reduces reperfusion, which can further exacerbate cerebral edema.

B is incorrect because it is appropriate to cover the cooling pad with a sheet to prevent skin damage.

C is incorrect because it is appropriate to keep the patient dry to prevent frostbite.

D is incorrect because it is appropriate to check skin condition before, during, and after using the cooling pad.

75. A new nursing graduate has written a plan of care for a child who has undergone tonsillectomy. The charge nurse assists with changing the plan of care if which of the following interventions is documented?

    A. Suction q 4 hours
    B. Offer clear liquids when awake
    C. Monitor for bleeding from tonsillectomy sites
    D. Eliminate dairy products from the diet

Rationale:

Correct answer: A

After a tonsillectomy procedure, suction equipment should be made available at the bedside but suctioning is not performed unless an airway obstruction occurs.

B is incorrect because cool, clear liquids are encouraged. (The nurse must also assess for pain, as a tonsillectomy procedure often requires pain control postoperatively.)

C is incorrect because monitoring for bleeding is important after any surgery.

D is incorrect because dairy products such as milk can coat the throat, increasing the need to clear the throat and increase risk for bleeding.

76. A patient on the medical floor has seizure precautions ordered. The RN reviews the care plan developed by the student nurse. The nurse will instruct the nursing student to remove which intervention?

A. Keep room lights on at night

B. Assist with ambulation

C. Monitor while showering

D. Keep bed in the lowest position

Rationale:

Correct answer: A

Seizure precautions require a quiet and restful environment. The patient should be allowed undisturbed sleep with a night light for safety.

B is incorrect because assisting the patient with ambulation is appropriate.

C is incorrect because the patient should be monitored during activities.

D is incorrect because the bed should be kept in the lowest position for safety.

(Note: Tips for seizure precautions: avoid flashing lights, alcohol, lack of sleep, hyperventilation, low blood sugar, and loud noises, which can trigger a seizure.)

77. The nurse is observing the unlicensed assistive personnel (UAP) caring for an elderly patient who had left hip pinning following a fall with left hip fracture five days ago. The nurse intervenes if the UAP does which of the following?

A. Leaves side rails down so the patient can get in and out of bed easily

B. Makes sure the night light works

C. Answers the call light quickly

D. Places the call light within reach

Rationale:

Correct answer: A

Patient safety is of the utmost importance, especially with patients who have a history of falls. The nurse should intervene if the UAP leaves the bed side rails down, as this could lead to a fall.

B is incorrect because working night lights are appropriate for patient safety.

C is incorrect because prompt answering of the call light could prevent a fall.

D is incorrect because leaving the call light within reach could prevent a fall.

78. The registered nurse is working with a nursing student caring for a 59-year-old patient being weaned from the ventilator using a T-piece. Which of the following is not part of the procedure of ventilator weaning with T-piece?

    A. Removing the patient from the ventilator for a short time
    B. Connecting the T-piece to the artificial airway
    C. Providing oxygen through the T-piece at a FiO2 10% higher than the ventilator setting
    D. Gradually decreasing ventilator respiratory rate until patient is performing all work of breathing

Rationale:

Correct answer: D

This describes synchronized intermittent mandatory ventilation (SIMV). In SIMV, the ventilator gives the patient a set number of breaths per minute at a specific tidal volume. The patient can breathe spontaneously between machine breaths. The ventilator senses the beginning of the patient's next spontaneous breath and synchronizes the machine breath with the patient's respiratory pattern. As the patient progressively increases the tidal volume of his spontaneous breaths, the machine can be set to deliver a lower number of breaths per minute.

A is incorrect because when weaning using the T-piece, the patient is removed from the ventilator for a short time, usually five minutes to begin with. The patient breathes humidified oxygen through the T-piece during the trial and then is placed back on the ventilator.

B is incorrect because the T-piece is connected to the artificial airway which is still in place in the patient's trachea.

C is incorrect because the FiO2 delivered with the T-piece is set 10% higher than the ventilator setting. Each subsequent trial lasts longer than the previous one as the patient's respiratory muscles become stronger and the patient increasingly tolerates breathing on their own. Once they can breathe spontaneously for two hours without clinical distress, they can be extubated.

79. The registered nurse is working with a new nursing graduate on the ICU. The nurse determines the new nursing graduate is competent to care for a patient on a ventilator when the new nurse does which of the following?

    A. Asks the respiratory therapist to routinely check the ventilator
    B. Calls the respiratory therapist when suction is needed
    C. Teaches family members to silence ventilator alarm when the patient coughs
    D. Allows the patient to rest after morning care

Rationale:

Correct answer: A

The respiratory therapist must routinely check and monitor the ventilator. The RT and the RN work together to manage the respiratory care of the patient on a ventilator.

B is incorrect because the RN can suction the patient on a ventilator without the assistance of the RT.

C is incorrect because family members should not be encouraged to touch the equipment. Alarms can be bothersome and noisy, but their purpose is to alert the nurse of potential complications. The alarm may be silenced by the RN or the RT when suctioning is performed but should be done cautiously after the RN has assessed the patient.

D is incorrect because it is appropriate for patient comfort, but not specific to caring for a patient on a ventilator.

80. The nursing student has developed a plan of care for a patient undergoing mastoidectomy. The RN intervenes and requests a revision if which of the following interventions is included?

   A. Assess for pain, dizziness, nausea
   B. Keep head of bed elevated 300
   C. Instruct the patient to lie on affected side to promote drainage
   D. Assess for cranial nerve VII injury

Rationale:

Correct answer: C

A mastoidectomy is a surgical procedure in which a portion of the mastoid bone is removed, usually after an ear infection that did not respond to medical treatment. Following a mastoidectomy, the patient should lie on the unaffected side to prevent swelling and pain, and the dressing should be assessed for drainage or bleeding.

A is incorrect because it is appropriate to assess for pain, dizziness, and nausea after a mastoidectomy.

B is incorrect because the head of bed should be kept elevated 30°.

D is incorrect because the patient should be assessed for cranial nerve VII (facial nerve) injury, which presents as complete or partial paralysis of the face. The nurse should assess for symmetry when asking the patient to raise both eyebrows, frown, show upper and lower teeth, close both eyes tightly, and puff out cheeks. Taste should also be assessed.

81. The nursing student is preparing to instruct a patient on administration of a new benzodiazepine anxiolytic. The RN intervenes if the student plans to include which of the following in the patient's instructions?

   A. Avoid driving or operating heavy machinery until alertness and response to medication is known
   B. Do not skip medication doses
   C. Double a dose if one is missed
   D. Do not use alcohol while taking the medication

Rationale:

Correct answer: C

The patient should be instructed to take the medication as prescribed, not to double up doses, and not to increase or stop taking the medication. Abrupt stopping of the medication could cause tremors, vomiting, nausea, and abdominal pain. Benzodiazepines include lorazepam, midazolam, diazepam, and chlordiazepoxide. They are used to treat anxiety, alcohol withdrawal, and seizures, and can be used as sedation.

A is incorrect because avoiding driving is an appropriate instruction. Benzodiazepines can cause lethargy, hangover, respiratory depression, and hypotension.

B is incorrect because avoiding skipping doses is an appropriate instruction. The medication should be taken as prescribed and not discontinued abruptly, because withdrawal can occur. These medications must be weaned off slowly.

D is incorrect because avoiding alcohol is an appropriate instruction because alcohol increases sedation when used with benzodiazepines.

82. The nurse manager of the telemetry unit is responsible for the number of healthcare staff reporting to them. What principle does this refer to?

   A. Span of control
   B. Unity of command
   C. Carrot and stick principle
   D. Esprit de corps

Rationale:

Correct answer: A

Span of control is the number of personnel who directly report to the nurse manager.

B is incorrect because unity of command is the concept that each employee is responsible to only one supervisor, who reports to another supervisor and so forth.

C is incorrect because the carrot and stick principle is not related to number of direct reports. This principle is characterized by the use of both rewards and punishments to induce cooperation. This principle is not effective for use in nursing leadership.

D is incorrect because esprit de corps is not related to number of direct reports. Esprit de corps is a sense of unity and common interests and responsibilities, as developed among a group of persons closely associated with a task or cause. This does not describe the relationship between a unit manager and the staff nurses.

83. The new nurse manager is learning about how to perform performance appraisals. Which of the following is not true regarding performance appraisal?

    A. Keeping staff members informed about specific impressions of their work can improve performance
    B. A verbal appraisal can substitute a written appraisal
    C. Patients are the best source for personnel appraisal
    D. Outcomes of performance appraisal rests with staff primarily

Rationale:

Correct answer: C

Patients can be a useful source of information about staff performance, but they don't possess the professional knowledge in order to be able to accurately evaluate nursing care or skills. Direct observation while performing patient care is the best source for performance appraisal.

A is incorrect because the statement is true.

B is incorrect because the statement is true.

D is incorrect because the statement is true.

84. The RN is caring for patients at a rehabilitation facility. A 72-year-old patient recovering from surgery to repair hip fracture asks the nurse about the purpose of a living will. Which is the appropriate response by the RN?

    A. "A living will tells us who you want us to call if you become confused and cannot make your own medical decisions."

B. "Your living will gives us details about your finances and how you want your personal belongings and assets divided, in the event of your death."

C. "A living will tells the healthcare team what your wishes are regarding your care."

D. "Because you are older than 70, it is strongly encouraged that you have a living will in your chart, so we can best care for you."

Rationale:

Correct answer: C

The living will indicates the patient's wishes for how they should be cared for in an emergency or if they become unable to communicate their wishes to the staff. Topics covered include resuscitation, desired quality of life, and end-of-life treatments including treatments the patient doesn't want to receive. This document advises the healthcare team how to approach patient treatment and ensures that the individual's medical wishes are honored.

A is incorrect because this statement describes a durable power of attorney (DPOA). The DPOA must never contradict the terms of the living will.

B is incorrect because a living will is used for health care purposes only. The DPOA will contain more information about who should receive the patient's belongings in the event of death.

D is incorrect because all adult patients should be encouraged to have a living will, not only the elderly.

Select All That Apply

85. The nurse manager is interested in improving hand-off communication on the nursing unit. Which of the following actions by the nurse manager would be best in achieving this goal? (Select all that apply):

    A. Coach and mentor the nurses as hand-off is performed
    B. Conduct hand-off audits
    C. Create a guide of topics that need to be included in hand-off
    D. Encourage questions during hand-off
    E. Award raises based on hand-off reporting compliance

Rationale:

Correct answer: A, B, C, D

Coaching and mentoring with nurse manager participation and observation of hand-off, as well as audits, reinforce quality. Standardizing hand-off with a guide will hard-wire the process and make it more effective. Encouraging staff questions also encourages critical thinking. These are all valid options for achieving the goal of hand-off communication improvement.

E is incorrect because raises should be earned based on multiple factors (such as job performance, attendance, length of employment, and patient satisfaction) not just one measure (hand-off communication compliance.)

86. The new nurse is interested in utilizing evidence-based practice (EBP) when caring for critical care patients. Which of the following factors does the nurse consider when planning care using EBP? (Select all that apply):

    A. Nurse's expertise
    B. Cost-saving methods
    C. Patient preferences
    D. Research findings
    E. Patient values

Rationale:

Correct answer: A, C, D, E

Evidence-based practice (EBP) is practice based on current evidence and research findings, patient preferences and values, as well as the nurse's expertise to provide the best care. These methods lead to improved patient outcomes.

B is incorrect because cost saving is not a focus of EBP.

87. The nurse manager is discussing goals of the department at a unit meeting. Which of the following choices are examples of nursing department goals? (Select all that apply):

    A. Reduce response time in emergencies to two minutes
    B. Increase patient satisfaction rate
    C. C. Increase nurse retention
    D. D. Eliminate delayed administration of antibiotics
    E. E. Establish rapport with patients

Rationale:

Correct answer: B, C

A goal is the result or achievement toward which effort is directed. Goals are statements that indicate desired results that unit or department efforts are directed toward. A goal is not a specific objective, but a statement about what the unit is aiming for.

A is incorrect because response time is a specific, measurable objective. An example of a goal under which this objective would fall is: "Improve nursing service delivery during code blue situations."

D is incorrect because eliminating delayed administration of antibiotics is an objective that can be tracked and measured. An example of a goal under which this objective would fall is: "Improve timeliness of medication administration."

E is incorrect because establishing patient rapport is a measurable objective for the goal of "Increase patient satisfaction rate."

88. The intensive care unit (ICU) charge nurse is making patient assignments. Which of the following patients is appropriate to assign to the telemetry nurse floated to the ICU for the day? (Select all that apply):

   A. Patient admitted for chest pain for whom myocardial infarction (MI) has been ruled out
   B. Ventilated patient requiring frequent repositioning, oral care, and who has a nitroprusside infusion
   C. Stable post-operative patient using a patient-controlled analgesia (PCA) pump
   D. Patient on the cardiac monitor displaying frequent dysrhythmias
   E. Patient on the intra-aortic balloon pump (IABP)

Rationale:

Correct answer: A, C, D

A telemetry nurse floated to the ICU can be assigned stable patients with diagnoses the telemetry nurse is familiar with and patients requiring procedures, medications, and equipment that the nurse is competent in delivering and utilizing. The telemetry nurse can care for the non-critical patient admitted for chest pain, a patient using a PCA pump, and the patient experiencing dysrhythmias.

B is incorrect because the telemetry nurse does not routinely care for ventilated patients. A continuous nitroprusside infusion is not commonly seen on a telemetry unit, so this patient needs an experienced ICU nurse who is familiar with the care of the ventilated patient and who is familiar with titrating this powerful vasodilator often used for shock, cardiac arrest, and anaphylaxis.

E is incorrect because the IABP patients require an experienced ICU nurse. The IABP is used to treat left ventricular failure or cardiogenic shock, is placed in the proximal descending aorta. The balloon is automatically inflated during diastole and deflated just prior to and during systole. The patient requires hourly pressure measurements and frequent neurovascular observation with Doppler. The nurse must be familiar with balloon pump waveform characteristics.

89. The new nurse has a six-month performance review with the nurse manager. Which of the following actions by the nurse manager is appropriate? (Select all that apply):

    A. The nurse manager asks another nurse to attend the review as a witness
    B. The nurse manager tells the nurse the review is manager-centered
    C. The review is private between the nurse and nurse manager
    D. The nurse manager tells the nursing staff about the review so another nurse can be asked to read the review
    E. The nurse manager identifies positive and negative characteristics of the nurse

Rationale:

Correct answer: C, E

A performance review is a private meeting between the nurse manager and the staff member and is designed to identify strengths and weaknesses of the staff member. Encouragement can be provided and opportunities to improve can be brought to the nurse's attention.

A is incorrect because a performance review is confidential between the nurse and the manager.

B is incorrect because a performance review is staff member centered.

D is incorrect because a performance review is confidential between the nurse and the manager and no other staff members will have privy to the documented review.

90. The nurse is working with an unlicensed assistive personnel (UAP) in caring for a group of patients. The nurse can delegate which of the following actions to the UAP? (Select all that apply):

    A. Ambulating a patient complaining of weakness to the bathroom
    B. Checking the blood glucose level of a patient on an insulin infusion
    C. Administrating acetaminophen 500 mg PO to a patient with a temperature of 99.7
    D. Assisting a chronic renal failure patient out of bed for transfer to the dialysis unit
    E. Notifying the healthcare provider of a patient complaining of unrelieved pain after opioid administration

Rationale:

Correct answer: A, B, D

The UAP is capable of performing many skills and procedures under the supervision of the nurse including ambulating a patient to the bathroom, checking blood glucose levels, and getting a patient out of bed. The nurse is responsible for providing information about the expecting results and findings when delegating and the nurse will inform the UAP under which circumstances the nurse should be contacted.

C is incorrect because UAP cannot administer medications.

E is incorrect because UAP do not communicate with the healthcare provider about patient findings, nor can the UAP take orders from the healthcare provider.

91. The charge nurse on the medical-surgical unit is making patient assignments. Which patients can the licensed practical nurse (LPN) be assigned to? (Select all that apply):

    A. Post-operative day two patient who needs a unit of blood
    B. Patient just admitted from the healthcare provider's office
    C. Patient who is NPO and has only intravenous (IV) medications
    D. Patient admitted for chest pain who may be discharged today
    E. Patient admitted from the assisted living center for urinary tract infection (UTI)

Rationale:

Correct answer: D, E

LPNs have different capabilities in each state depending on the nursing state regulatory body and training or certification. In general, LPNs can care for stable patients, administer medications, and provide basic care to patients whose outcomes are predictable and are not suffering unexplained symptoms.

A is incorrect because administration of blood products requires the RN. Each U.S. state board of nursing designates what specific activities the LPN can and cannot do, but for the NCLEX, the LPN cannot administer blood or blood products because this not a task that is delegated to LPNs across all 50 states. (However, in an emergency case, the LPN CAN stop a blood transfusion.)

B is incorrect because the RN must care for the newly admitted patient. The LPN cannot perform the comprehensive initial assessment.

C is incorrect because the LPN cannot administer IV push medications.

92. A new nurse on the cardiac unit notifies the charge nurse another nurse has been harassing and bullying her, especially when she makes a mistake. Which of the following initial actions by the charge nurse is appropriate? (Select all that apply):

A. Reassure the new nurse it will improve with time and that this a common experience as a new graduate.

B. Ask the new nurse to explain more about the problem.

C. Facilitate a discussion between the new nurse and the experienced nurse.

D. Notify the nurse manager of the bullying problem.

E. Suggest the new nurse tell the experienced nurse to discuss how the bullying impacts her practice.

Rationale:

Correct answer: B, C, E

Bullying by nurses is a problem in many healthcare facilities. It is important to identify the behavior, discuss it with the nurse bully, and attempt to find ways to stop it. It is appropriate for the charge nurse to talk to the experienced nurse who is bullying the new nurse, facilitate a discussion between the two, and suggest the new nurse discuss the impact of the bullying on her practice.

A is incorrect because this statement dismisses the concern that has been verbalized by the new nurse. Bullying and harassment should not be ignored as they can negatively impact job performance, job satisfaction, retention of nursing staff, and patient outcomes.

D is incorrect because it is the charge nurse's role to handle this type of interpersonal conflict in the unit. The nurse manager does not need to initially get involved with the problem unless the two nurses, along with the charge nurse, are unable to come to a solution.

93. The charge nurse is making assignments for the oncology unit and needs to place a new unlicensed assistive personnel (UAP) with a nurse preceptor. Which of the following nurses would be appropriate to pair the new UAP with for the shift? (Select all that apply):

A. New graduate nurse who just came off orientation

B. Experienced nurse who loves teaching

C. Float nurse who has been assigned to the unit for the shift

D. Nurse who has a couple of years of experience and was once an UAP

E. An experienced UAP

Rationale:

Correct answer: B, D

Precepting of a new UAP must be done by an experienced RN who knows the unit well. The UAP will need to be trained about unit policies, location of equipment (crash cart, linens, meal trays, medical supplies, bathroom, sharps disposal bins, fire extinguishers).

The RN will also be responsible for evaluating the ability of the UAP to perform tasks (such as blood glucose testing, vital sign measurement, transferring patients to bed/chair, repositioning, bathing, ambulating). Those who love to teach and were once UAPs make excellent preceptors for new UAPs.

A is incorrect because a new graduate nurse is still mastering time management skills and is unable to precept yet. The new RN should not be assigned any extraneous tasks or obligations while initially working to become comfortable with the daily routine, workload, and flow of the unit. This is often a period of six months or longer.

C is incorrect because the float nurse is not necessarily familiar with the unit and may not be appropriate to precept a UAP on this unit.

E is incorrect because the requirement is for the UAP to be placed with a nurse preceptor. An experienced UAP will be a peer source of support to the new UAP but cannot be delegated the responsibility to train a new UAP.

94. The emergency room nurse is caring for a patient with assistance from the unlicensed assistive personnel (UAP). Which of the following tasks can the nurse delegate to the UAP? (Select all that apply):

    A. Apply a sling to the patient with a dislocated shoulder
    B. Draw blood samples for lab testing
    C. Insert a peripheral IV
    D. Transfer a patient via stretcher to the medical-surgical unit
    E. Teach a patient how to care for stitches

Rationale:

Correct answer: A, D

The emergency room UAP can perform many tasks under the supervision of the nurse. These tasks include applying slings and splints and transferring a patient to the inpatient unit (If cardiac monitoring is required, the RN must accompany the patient during the transfer.) The nurse can delegate all of these tasks to the UAP. The RN should not delegate patient education, nursing decisions, sterile procedures, or highly technical tasks.

C is incorrect because insertion of a peripheral IV requires RN assessment and evaluation.

E is incorrect because the RN is the only member of the nursing team who can perform patient education.

95. The nurse caring for patients on the intensive care unit (ICU) is feeling overwhelmed with the patient assignment three hours into the shift. Which of the following actions would be most appropriate for the nurse to perform? (Select all that apply):

    A. Alert the charge nurse that the patient assignment is too much, and request a change
    B. Alert the charge nurse and ask for help
    C. Talk to another nurse about how heavy the patient assignment is
    D. Delegate tasks to the unlicensed assistive personnel (UAP) and another nurse
    E. Notify the nursing supervisor

Rationale:

Correct answer: B, D

Patient assignments can be overwhelming at times, depending on patient acuity and patient status. Nurses should always go up the chain of command and request help when feeling overwhelmed. Delegation of tasks to other members of the nursing team (LPN/LVN, UAP) is also appropriate. These are the most appropriate actions to prevent mistakes and increase patient safety.

A is incorrect because the charge nurse should be notified but requesting a change in assignments is inappropriate. The charge nurse should be able to assist the RN with care of the patients and help utilize support staff such as LPN/LVN and UAP to decrease workload on the RN.

C is incorrect because each nurse is responsible for their own patient assignment and any issues with workload should be addressed up the chain of command, not with peers.

E is incorrect because it is the charge nurse's role to handle this type of assignment/workload difficulty. The nurse manager does not need to initially get involved with the problem unless the assigned RN and charge nurse are unable to come to a solution.

96. The healthcare provider is yelling at a nurse for not being able to answer a question regarding a patient who is not part of the nurse's assignment. Which interventions would be most appropriate by the charge nurse? (Select all that apply):

    A. Ask the healthcare provider to stop yelling at the nurse
    B. Facilitate a discussion between the healthcare provider and the nurse
    C. Ask the nurse what occurred to cause the healthcare provider to yell
    D. Have the nurse step away and talk to the healthcare provider about the reaction privately
    E. Tell the nurse the healthcare provider is known for reacting inappropriately

Rationale:4

Correct answer: A, B, D

Confrontation may be useful in identifying the problem and proposing a solution. When a healthcare provider yells at a nurse inappropriately, it is always appropriate for the charge nurse to intervene, and advocate for the nurse. Facilitated discussion may be necessary to help the provider understand that the RN does not yet know about the patient. The charge nurse may also talk to the healthcare provider in private about the reaction.

C is incorrect because it places blame on the new nurse and avoids confrontation with the healthcare provider.

E is incorrect because it is dismissive and validates the healthcare provider's inappropriate behavior. The charge nurse should not avoid problems.

97. The nurse is working with the new unlicensed assistive personnel (UAP), planning to perform a bed bath on a comatose patient with a sacral decubitus stage II ulcer. The nurse directs the UAP do which of the following? (Select all that apply):

   A. Obtain blood specimen tubes and place at the bedside
   B. Ensure that disposable gloves are available at the bedside
   C. Open the curtains to allow sunlight in to stimulate the patient during the procedure
   D. Remove the top sheet and blanket and place it in the soiled laundry bin as the bed bath begins
   E. Wash the perineum last, avoiding contact with the ulcer dressing

Rationale:

Correct answer: B, E

Disposable gloves are required when performing a bed bath because the nursing team may come into contact with bodily fluids. The perineal area is the last body area to be washed when performing a bed bath. The nurse will perform the decubitus ulcer dressing change with or without the assistance of the UAP, but the nurse remains responsible for the dressing change and for assessing the ulcer when the old dressing is removed.

A is incorrect because blood specimen tubes are not necessary equipment for performing either a bed bath or a decubitus ulcer dressing change.

C is incorrect because curtains should be closed during a bed bath to maintain patient privacy. The curtains can be opened to allow sunlight into the room after the bath is completed and the patient is covered.

D is incorrect because the blanket should not be completely removed at the beginning of the procedure. The nurse and UAP should uncover the top portion of the patient's body to begin the bath and then cover the patient with a clean sheet before completely removing the blanket to bathe the lower portion of the body. This provides for both warmth and privacy.

98. The nurse is working with a new nursing graduate who is preparing to irrigate an adult patient's right ear due to buildup of cerumen. Which action by the new nursing graduate indicates the nurse needs to provide more education regarding this procedure? (Select all that apply):

    A. The patient is positioned with the right ear facing up
    B. The irrigating solution is warmed to body temperature
    C. The new nurse directs the irrigation solution directly toward the tympanic membrane
    D. The new nurse gently pulls the pinna down and back before irrigating
    E. The patient is positioned with the right ear facing down after irrigation

Rationale:

Correct answer: A, C

The patient should be sitting up or lying down with the head tilted toward the side of the affected ear. (The affected ear should not be facing up, as this does not facilitate drainage of fluid and cerumen out of the ear.) The patient or another staff member should hold a basin under the ear to receive the irrigating solution. The auditory canal can be straightened by pulling the pinna up and back for an adult. The irrigating solution should be directed at the roof of the ear canal to prevent injury to the tympanic membrane. Continuous flow of the solution in and out of the ear prevents increased pressure in the canal which can be painful.

B is incorrect (does not indicate need for more education) because it is appropriate to warm the irrigation solution to body temperature.

D is incorrect (does not indicate need for more education) because this is the appropriate method for straightening the ear canal. This helps the solution to reach all areas of the ear more easily. (Pull the pinna down and back to straighten the ear canal for an infant).

E is incorrect (does not indicate need for more education) because it is appropriate to face the irrigated side down to allow for excess solution to exit the ear.

99. The registered nurse (RN) is supervising the care of a patient with acquired immunodeficiency syndrome (AIDS). The new licensed practical nurse (LPN) is preparing to suction the patient. The RN determines the procedure will be performed safely when the LPN selects which of the following personal protective equipment (PPE)? (Select all that apply):

A. Gloves

B. Mask

C. Protective eyewear

D. Respirator

E. Gown

Rationale:

Correct answer: A, B, C

It is the responsibility of the RN to ensure a new LPN delivers patient care safely and maintains patient safety while following procedural guidelines. Caring for a patient with AIDS requires the use of standard precautions, including wearing gloves, mask, and protective eyewear when suctioning the patient.

D is incorrect because a respirator mask is worn by healthcare providers when caring for a patient with airborne precautions. AIDS requires standard precautions.

E is incorrect because a gown is only necessary when a large amount of body fluid or blood contact is anticipated.

100. The registered nurse (RN) is working with a new graduate nurse caring for a patient on the cardiac floor. The RN determines the new nurse is practicing medication administration safely when the new nurse does which of the following? (Select all that apply):

A. Verifies patient by two patient identifiers

B. States the indications and monitoring parameters for which medications are administered

C. Checks pulse rate before administration of a beta-blocker

D. Documents the medications in the nurse's notes

E. Administers IV fluids without an IV pump

Rationale:

Correct answer: A, B, C

The safely practicing new graduate nurse will use two patient identifiers, know the indications and monitoring parameters for medications, and check vital signs including pulse rate before beta-blockers and medications that affect heart rate and blood pressure are administered.

D is incorrect because medications are documented in the medication administration record (MAR).

E is incorrect because IV fluids should be administered with an IV pump to prevent fluid overload. The exception is in an emergency when a large amount of fluid (bolus) needs to be delivered quickly.

We hope you have enjoyed this guide! We can't wait to hear about your success with the NCLEX-RN Exam. Please leave a review wherever you bought the book and share your success.

From the creators at,
NurseEdu.com

Made in the USA
Columbia, SC
03 March 2023

13310651R00128